100
Ways to Stay
Young

100
Ways to Stay Young

Great tips and treatments for diet, lifestyle, health, and beauty

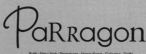

Bath · New York · Singapore · Hong Kong · Cologne · Delhi
Melbourne · Amsterdam · Johannesburg · Auckland · Shenzhen

First published by Parragon in 2011

Parragon
Queen Street House
4 Queen Street
Bath, BA1 1HE
www.parragon.com

ISBN: 978-1-4454-5226-5

Produced by Guy Croton

Note: The authors and publishers disclaim any
liability, loss, injury, or damage incurred as a
consequence, directly or indirectly, of the use
and application of the contents of this book.

See page 224 for photograph copyright details

Cover images:
Front cover images L-R:
Oranges and leaves © istockphoto
Yoga mat © istockphoto
Cup of green tea © istockphoto

Back cover images:
Woman in athletic gear © Jamie Grill/
Getty Images
Strawberries and blueberries © istockphoto

Printed in China

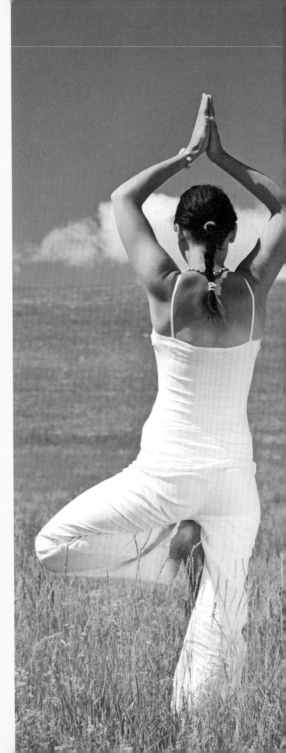

Contents

Introduction

Staying young, remaining as youthful as possible for as long as possible, has been a preoccupation of men and women since the dawn of time. Unfortunately we all age—it's part of the human condition—but there is a great deal you can do to delay the process and feel good about yourself as you do so.

FEEL YOUR WAY

In fact, how you feel is half the battle. The age you are at any time in your life is not especially important—it is how old you feel inside that counts. The years roll by and the number that you are labeled with gradually accumulates, but we all age at different rates and we all have different experiences in our lives. There really are no guaranteed certainties about aging—or staying young—it is all about how you feel and cope personally.

PLAN TO STAY YOUNG

Part of feeling young and remaining so for as long as possible involves making a conscious decision to make the most of life as you get older—to live it to the full. Staying active and healthy for as long as you can is a big part of this, and we show you countless ways of doing this throughout this book. However, setting goals and planning your future will help you in your objective. What do you want to do with your life as you become older? Maybe you want to travel; perhaps you want to spend more time with your children or grandchildren; you might even want to embark on a new career. The choice is yours, but it will pay to have some notion of where you are taking your life as you get older and will motivate you in the process of endeavoring to stay young.

THE RIGHT DIET

One of the most important things you can do in your quest for youthfulness is to eat a healthy diet. This is probably the key factor in your general health throughout your life. We are still learning about how various foods affect our bodies and minds and the precise nutritional value of much of what we eat—new scientific findings and revelations are announced every day—but what is indisputable is that a balanced diet full of foods that have a high nutritional value will benefit you whoever you are and whatever age you might have attained.

The "right diet" involves a balance of the five key food groups—protein, carbohydrates, fiber, fats, and sugars—and we give you comprehensive information about how to achieve this balance in Chapter 1, "Food for life." The most important thing is to ensure that you eat a sufficient number of "good" foods every day, while avoiding foods high in unhealthy sugars and saturated fats that wear down the body, increase blood pressure, and contribute to the likelihood of heart disease.

Eating to stay young need not be a chore—there are lots of truly delicious and enjoyable foods that you can make part of your regular diet while benefiting your health. These are covered in detail in the following pages. The really good news is that some of the very best anti-aging foods are actually regarded as treats and luxuries in many societies. These include red wine and dark chocolate, which are both full of health-giving antioxidants that are particularly beneficial as we become older. Having said that, as with most things in life, balance is the key. A little of what you fancy might not do you any harm, but too much will put your caloric balance out of kilter and might result in you seeing inches added to your waistline.

EXERCISE FOR LIFE

For many of us, exercise was something that we were obliged to do at school in gym classes once or twice a week. It was often cold, uncomfortable, and not particularly enjoyable. However, exercise has come a long way since then. These days there is a multitude of choices available and exercise facilities have generally become far more sophisticated and user-friendly.

These developments reflect an ever-growing understanding of the benefits of exercise to human health. Again, whatever age you are and whatever your physical condition, a little regular exercise will benefit your general health and make you feel—and probably look—younger.

Get in the habit of doing a little exercise—make it part of your weekly routine—and you will soon reap the rewards and maybe even begin to enjoy it. There are so many different things you could do! If you don't fancy sweating in a gym surrounded by other people, buy an exercise bike or a rowing machine to use in the privacy of your own home. If you don't like the idea of working out with machines, take up running, swimming, or racquet sports, such as badminton or tennis. If these sound too strenuous, simply make a brisk walk or some gardening part of your daily routine. All these things and more will improve your health and help keep you young—and their benefits are covered in detail throughout Chapter 2, "Fit mind, fit body."

KEEP YOUR MIND SHARP

While bodily fitness is of undoubted importance as we become older, keeping your brain in good shape and your mind sharp is of equal significance. One of the unfortunate by-products of aging is a decline in mental acuity. Many people become aware of problems, such as forgetfulness, vagueness, and mental fatigue, as they become older, symptoms that if left unchecked can ultimately result in dementia or Alzheimer's disease. However, the good news is that much can be done not only to slow this process down but to reverse it altogether.

Whereas scientists used to believe that we are born with a finite number of brain cells that begin dying out from about the age of seven years, recent research indicates that we can in fact generate new cells into old age—and that this process of regeneration can be enhanced by our thinking and an increased degree of mental activity as we become older. It need not take much effort—simply reading books on a regular basis, doing crosswords, or su doku puzzles, or playing chess—all of these things will improve your mental sharpness and keep you feeling on top of things. Again, plenty of exercise and a moderate intake of alcohol and fatty foods will also help in this regard.

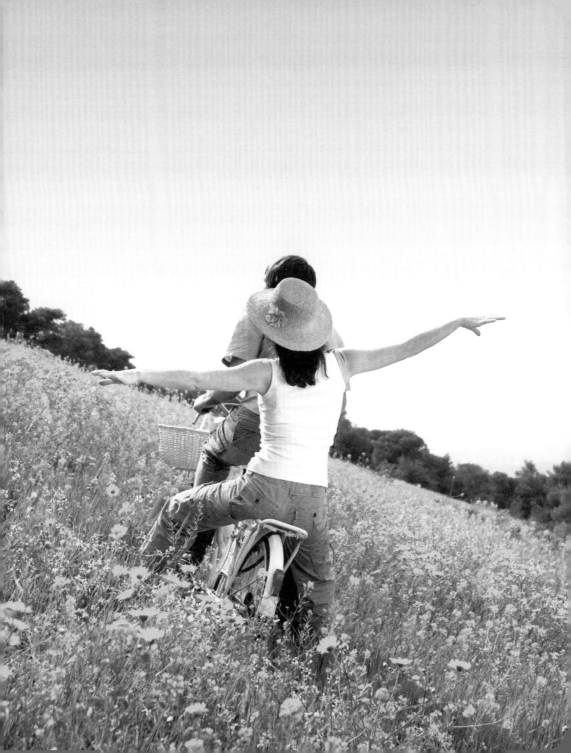

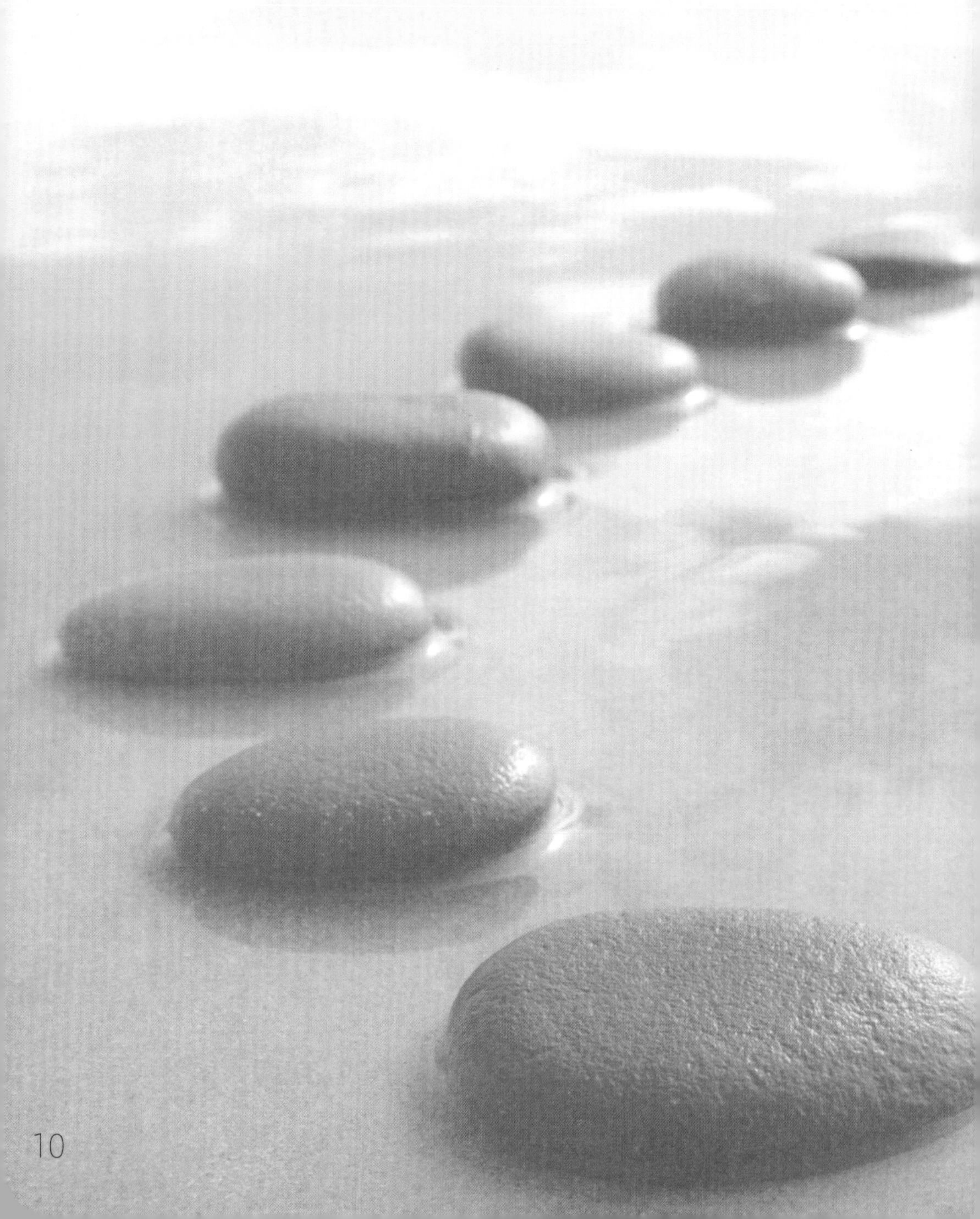

THINK POSITIVE

Another commonplace mental aspect of aging is a tendency to think negatively and to experience feelings of lower self-esteem. It can be easy to fall into this trap. As many people get older, they become less active, interact with fewer people, have fewer pastimes, and generally withdraw from areas of everyday life. This can begin a destructive cycle of self-doubt and worry— possibly even fear and loathing—which in turn can take its toll on the body and increase the aging process that is probably responsible for this general change of heart and mind in the first place.

To avoid this happening to you, it is vital to maintain a positive frame of mind and an enthusiastic, healthy approach to life. Why should you not feel as upbeat about things as you did when you were younger? Maybe it's because you feel that you have "let yourself go" a little and are no longer as attractive as you once were? If that is the case, turn to Chapter 3, "Focus on the face." This section of the book is packed with beauty tips and techniques that will help to rejuvenate your facial skin and looks and leave you feeling years younger.

But making physical fixes is only half the battle—you have got to believe in yourself and keep your mind going properly as well. Your thoughts have an incredible power over your life and dictate so much of how you live it. Learn how to maintain a positive and enthusiastic attitude toward your life and reap the rewards. Bear in mind what the great car magnate Henry Ford once said: "Whether you believe you can do a thing or not, you are right."

MIX YOUNG, STAY YOUNG

One of the most effective ways to keep yourself consistently feeling young is to spend a lot of time around younger people. The energy, enthusiasm, and general liveliness of the young tends to be highly infectious, so if you have young children or grandchildren, get out in the backyard or park with them and rediscover your own youthful energy and lust for life. Kids are always on the move, and their movement will keep you going, too. When it comes to aging, perhaps the most important piece of advice to keep in mind is "do not congeal." Stay active, stay mobile, stay young—it really does work.

If you spend a lot of time with young people, you might be self-conscious about how you look compared with them. If so, turn to Chapter 4, "Natural beauty." It is full of great tips on how to keep your skin, hair, and body looking young, fit, and vital the natural way. It will boost your confidence and stop you from feeling inferior to your younger companions in any way at all.

GET IN TOUCH WITH NATURE

If you are beginning to feel old and tired, it is so easy just to collapse on the couch and become a layabout. However, this is about the worst thing you can do. An endless diet of sitting in front of the television eating snacks and sipping drinks will simply accelerate your aging process and leave you feeling even lower on energy, drive, and enthusiasm than ever before.

So much better, instead, to head for the great outdoors! Nature is rejuvenating and will automatically make you feel more alive. Your body and mind deteriorate when they are idle, but out in the fresh air and sunshine, surrounded by the sounds, smells, and other stimuli of nature, they will come alive and will feel vital and invigorated once more.

It is impossible to overstate just how much good getting out and getting active will do you. Even if it is just a walk in the local woods, your health will benefit. Make it a cycle ride, a hike, or a camping trip, and the years will fall off you. Become a fresh air fanatic and start to feel younger right away.

THE MIND/BODY BALANCE

One of the intriguing things about how the human body works and ages is the extent to which it is reliant upon the state of the mind—and vice versa. This essential correlation is known as the "mind/body balance" and an analysis of its importance to the business of staying young is at the heart of Chapter 5, "Young on the inside." Look after your mind and you look after your body; take care of your physical health and you benefit your brain—it's really as simple as that. However this happy equilibrium is achieved, it will improve your chances of living longer in a healthier, better way.

There are so many positive things you can do to ensure that your mind/body balance remains healthy as you become older. You could laugh a lot, for a start. Laughing releases positive hormones and chemicals in the brain that will make you feel better—as well as those around you. Everybody loves someone with a sense of humor—whatever their age. You could take up new hobbies—for both the body and the mind. This might increase your level of social interaction, which will benefit you in a multitude of ways.

As you age—inevitably, unfortunately—be thankful for what you have and what you are. Your experience and knowledge count for a lot and make you who you are. An awareness of your uniqueness—in the form of a healthy self-regard, rather than any kind of arrogance—will stand you in good stead as the years pass, making you feel as young as possible, whichever road your life travels. Here's to a long, healthy, and happy life! Stay young!

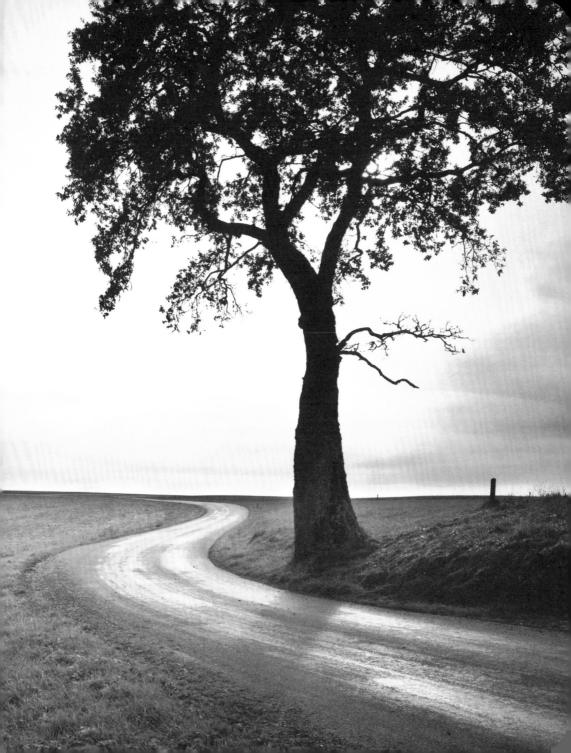

Food for life

Eating well is important throughout life and is central to remaining healthy and feeling youthful. The key is a balanced diet made up of foods that provide plenty of energy and satisfaction without overloading or damaging your body. This chapter offers tips on the best foods to eat, what to avoid, and how to control and monitor your diet, as well as one or two mouthwatering recipes that will keep you feeling well nourished, fit, and young.

Introduction

"You are what you eat," or so the old saying goes. As scientific research reveals more and more about our bodies and the nutritional value of foods, there would appear to be a great deal of truth in this statement. One thing is for sure: What you eat will have a great bearing on how young you look and feel.

EATING FOR YOUTHFULNESS

You eat primarily to stay alive, but making conscious choices about what you eat and how you eat it can have a hugely beneficial effect on your health and appearance as well as simply sustaining you. It is mainly nutrition, not the fact of aging itself, that determines the body's internal chemistry, and that chemistry determines, in large part, the quality and resilience of virtually every organ, cell, and system in the body. Consequently, everything from the condition of your skin to the quality of your bones, brain, and connective tissue is determined in part by what you eat. As a result, your eating habits are a major determinant in how quickly you begin to see and feel the effects of aging. Naturally, then, the better you eat the better you will look and feel.

EATING REALISTICALLY

While this chapter is full of great advice about what and how to eat in order to stay feeling young, we acknowledge that you are only human and that consequently it is not always easy to stick to a balanced, healthy diet—the straight and narrow of eating. However, if you observe these basic rules on top of the detailed advice in the following pages, you won't go far wrong:

- Avoid transfats, found in fast foods and products advertising hydrogenated oils—these cause internal inflammation, lead to the body's inability to regenerate organs, and will shorten your longevity.
- Avoid too much sugar—the body is unable to break down large amounts of sugars and in the process makes you look older by creating wrinkles.
- Avoid carbohydrate overload—similar to sugar, excess carbohydrates stress the body. This can age the body by leading to type 2 diabetes, metabolic syndrome, and heart disease.
- Avoid waiting to eat until you are starving—the hormone ghrelin is released when your brain senses it's hungry. It can take 30 minutes to normalize your ghrelin levels. This can trigger overeating and lead to obesity.
- Avoid eating when stressed—cortisol, a stress hormone, can prevent digestion; impact the stomach's acidity levels, preventing nutrient absorption; and make you more apt to make unhealthy food choices and overeat.

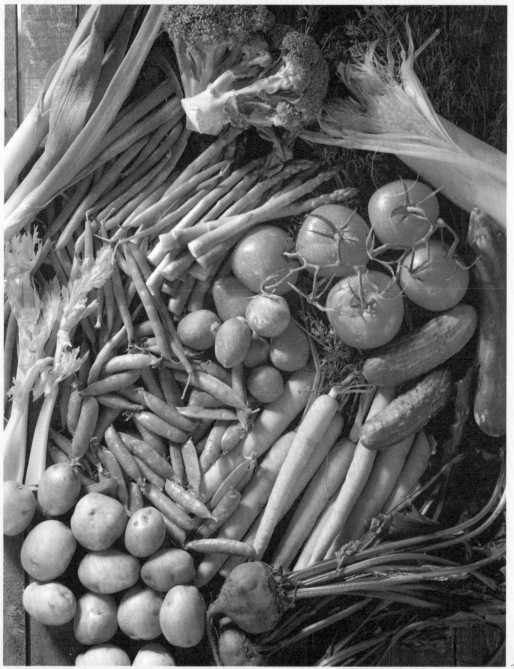

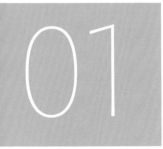

01

The importance of breakfast

Breakfast is the most important meal of the day. It follows the longest period of time you would normally go without eating, after several hours of sleep, and its name means to end a period of fasting, or not eating. Follow the advice here to get the most out of this essential meal.

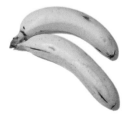

WHY EAT BREAKFAST?

You would not consider starting a long journey in your car without first filling it with fuel. By the same token, you should not begin a day without giving your body the sustenance it requires. Energy levels are low in the mornings, and your body needs an energy boost, in the form of food, to jump-start the day.

In our busy modern lives, breakfast is often grabbed in passing as an afterthought or even skipped altogether. This is not wise, because eating a healthy, balanced breakfast can have a really positive effect both physically and mentally.

THE BENEFITS OF BREAKFAST

A number of studies have shown that eating breakfast regularly leads to improved mood and better memory. Breakfast eaters also tend to be less stressed and feel calmer. Adults perform better in mental tasks after eating breakfast, and children who eat breakfast perform better in school.

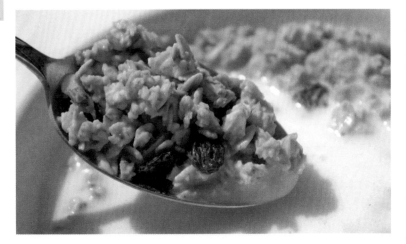

RIGHT Ideally your breakfast should include some form of whole grains—perhaps from a muesli or crunchy cereal, like the one shown here.

TOP BREAKFAST HINTS

- Aim to eat a breakfast that is high in carbohydrates and low in fat and sugar.

- Breakfast cereals are almost all fortified with minerals and vitamins, so along with lowfat milk, these provide a nutritious, balanced meal.

- If you prefer toast in the mornings, there are lots of different types of bread to choose from, for example: whole wheat; whole grain; bagels; rye bread.

- If you enjoy a cooked breakfast, you can make these healthier, by broiling instead of frying bacon or sausages.

- For a light breakfast, opt for lowfat yogurt with fresh or dried fruit.

- Breakfast provides an ideal opportunity to count toward your five daily servings of fruit and vegetables. A glass of fruit juice provides a useful source of vitamin C, as does adding dried fruit to breakfast cereals.

Breakfast should ideally provide around one-quarter of your daily nutritional requirements. Skipping breakfast, whether due to lack of time or trying to lose weight, can mean missing out on essential nutrients, and studies have shown that those who don't eat breakfast are unlikely to make up for these losses later in the day. This can have a negative effect on both short- and long-term health and can accelerate the aging process.

BELOW Breakfast is a good time to start the accumulation of your "five a day," with a couple portions of fruit or fruit juice.

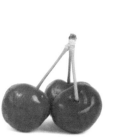
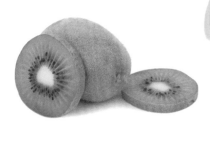

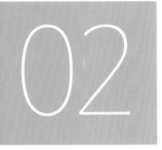

Drink plenty of water

In order for your skin to looks its best and most youthful, it is vital to remain well hydrated at all times. This means drinking lots of fresh, pure, cold water throughout the day. It doesn't have to be mineral water—water from the faucet will do just as well. Drinking water offers lots of other benefits, too.

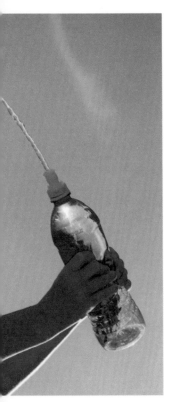

WHY IS WATER SO GOOD FOR YOU?

Water is the essence of human life. For a start, our bodies are made up of about 60 to 70 percent of water. Blood is mostly water, and your muscles, lungs, and brain all contain a lot of water. Your body needs water to regulate body temperature and to provide the means for nutrients to travel to all your organs. Water also transports oxygen to your cells, removes waste, and protects your joints and organs.

GETTING THE WATER HABIT

We are all encouraged to drink a lot of water from an early age, but very few people form the habit of drinking it regularly. If we don't drink enough water, we become dehydrated, which is bad for health and accelerates the aging process.

WATER AND WEIGHT LOSS

Water is a great tool for weight loss, not least because it often replaces high-calorie drinks, such as sodas or alcohol, with a drink that doesn't have any calories. It is also a great appetite suppressant.

WATER FOR HEALTHY SKIN

Drinking water can clear up your skin and keep it looking young and fresh. Many people often report a healthy glow after drinking a lot of fresh water.

ABOVE It is a good idea to take a bottle of fresh water with you wherever you go, particularly if you are exercising.

OTHER BENEFITS OF DRINKING WATER

• Being dehydrated can sap your energy and make you feel tired—even mild dehydration of as little as one or two percent of your body weight. If you are thirsty, you are already dehydrated—and this can lead to fatigue, muscle weakness, dizziness, and other symptoms.

• Another symptom of dehydration is headaches. In fact, often when we have headaches it is simply due to not drinking enough water. There are a lot of other causes of headaches, of course, but dehydration is one of the most common.

• Our digestive systems need a good amount of water to digest food properly. Often water can help cure stomach acid problems, and water combined with fiber can cure constipation, which is often a result of dehydration.

• The body uses water to help flush out toxins and waste products. Water literally cleanses the system and rids it of threatening elements.

• Drinking a healthy amount of water has also been found to reduce the risk of colon cancer by 45 percent. Drinking a lot of water can also reduce the risk of bladder cancer—by as much as 50 percent—and can potentially reduce the risk of breast cancer.

> ✳ TIP BOX
>
> **CUT YOUR HEART RISK**
> Drinking lots of water could lower your risk of a heart attack. Studies show that those who drink more than five glasses of water a day are 41 percent less likely to have one.

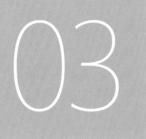

03

Eat more starchy foods

Starchy foods—technically known as "carbohydrates"—make up the food group that is your body's main source of energy. This group includes bread, pasta, rice, potatoes, noodles, cereals, and other starchy carbohydrates. These foods represent a vital component of a healthy, balanced diet.

HOW DO STARCHY FOODS HELP YOU STAY YOUNG?

With the exception of potatoes, the foods listed above are all produced from grains, such as wheat, corn, or rice. Grains can come in two forms—unrefined (often known as whole grains) or refined.

Unrefined or whole-grain forms provide far more nutrients than their refined counterparts, because they have not been stripped of their outer bran coating and inner germ during the milling process. Whole grains are rich in phytochemicals and antioxidants, which help to protect against coronary heart disease, certain cancers, and diabetes. Studies have shown that people who eat more whole grains tend to have a healthier heart, are generally fitter, and live longer.

* TIP BOX

READ THE LABEL
Nearly all foods now come with labels that provide details of their nutritional value. Choose products that specify that whole grains have been used in their production, as opposed to refined.

RIGHT & OPPOSITE
Unrefined wheat (right) and barley (opposite) are part of nature's treasure trove of starchy, fibrous foods, which should ideally form at least one-third of your daily diet.

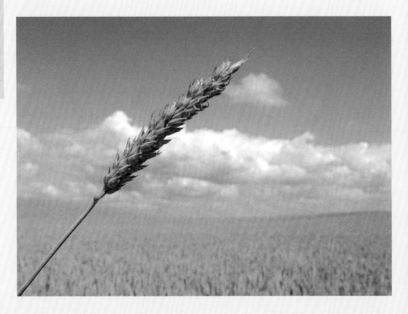

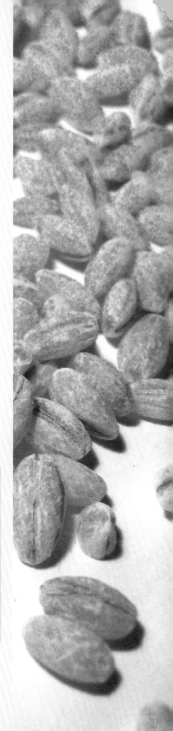

GO FOR WHOLE GRAINS

Whole grains should be a part of all meals, filling about a third of your plate. Most people get their whole-grain from whole-wheat bread or whole-grain breakfast cereals such as oatmeal, muesli, or whole-wheat cereals. Choose a whole-grain type over processed or refined grains, and look out for added sugar or salt.

Other whole grains include:
- Wheat
- Oats
- Barley
- Rye
- Corn.

Refined grains include white rice, white bread, and white pasta. While these can be beneficial as part of a balanced diet, they are not nearly as good for you as whole grains.

THE IMPORTANCE OF FIBER

Dietary fiber is found in plant foods (fruit, vegetables, and whole grains) and is essential for maintaining a healthy digestive system. Fiber cannot be fully digested and for this reason is often called bulk or roughage. The two types of fiber found in food are soluble and insoluble.

WHY IS FIBER GOOD FOR YOU?

- High-fiber foods take longer to digest, so they keep you feeling fuller for longer.

- Fiber helps in the digestive process and can help lower blood cholesterol.

- Fiber promotes bowel regularity and keeps the gastrointestinal tract clean.

- A high-fiber diet may help reduce the risk of developing diabetes and colorectal cancer.

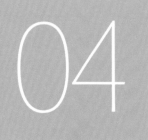

04

Eat more fruit & vegetables

A healthy diet includes eating at least five portions, and ideally more, of a variety of fruit or vegetables each day. Fruit and vegetables include fresh, frozen, canned, or dried types, as well as fruit juice. As a general rule, people who eat a lot of fruit and vegetables tend to be healthier and live longer.

ENJOY THE HEALTH BENEFITS

If you regularly eat a good amount of fresh fruit and vegetables, you have a lower chance of developing cardiovascular diseases due to hardening of the arteries (atheroma) and, thereby, significantly reduce your risk of having a heart attack or stroke. This particularly applies as you become older. Similarly, by eating lots of fruit and vegetables, you are less likely to develop some cancers, such as bowel and lung cancer.

Other benefits of fruit and vegetables are that they:

- Contain lots of fiber, which helps to keep your bowels healthy. Problems such as constipation and diverticular disease, are less likely to develop.
- Contain plenty of vitamins and minerals, which will keep you healthy.
- Are naturally low in fat.
- Are filling but are low in calories, so are a useful part of any weight-loss or diet plan.

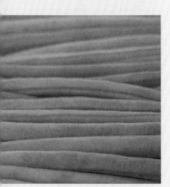

ABOVE Green beans are an excellent source of vitamin K, which is very important for bone health and prevents bone damage in older people.

WHAT IS A "PORTION" OF FRUIT OR VEGETABLES?

One portion of fruit or vegetables is roughly equivalent to:

- **One large fruit, such as an apple, pear, banana, orange or melon**

- **Two smaller fruits, such as plums, kiwis, satsumas, or clementines**

- **One cup of small fruits such as grapes, strawberries, or raspberries**

- **One glass of fresh fruit juice (5 fl oz)**

- **A normal portion of any vegetable (about two tablespoons).**

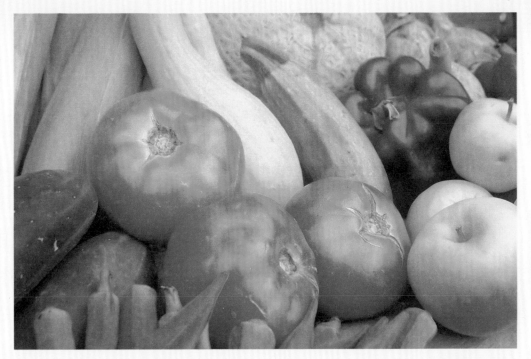

HOW DO FRUIT & VEGETABLES KEEP YOU YOUNG?

These foods are rich in vitamins and minerals that keep the body healthy. They also contain chemicals called antioxidants, such as carotene, which are thought to protect against damaging chemicals ("free radicals") that get into the body. Regular consumption of fresh fruit and vegetables will keep your bones, teeth, and organs healthy and will improve the look of your skin. Basically, this is how they contribute to keeping you looking and feeling young, although the exact way in which they prevent disease is not fully understood.

ABOVE Your "five a day" intake of fruit and vegetables should ideally comprise a range of as many different colors and textures as possible.

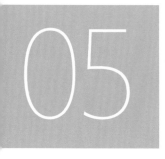

Follow the MUFA rule

Forget simplistic fat-free dieting. As an anti-aging food, monounsaturated fatty acids—MUFAs for short—are top of the list. Include a MUFA in every meal, especially if you are trying to lose weight, and use them as healthy snacks, too. These foods will keep you looking and feeling younger.

WHAT ARE THE BENEFITS?

MUFAs are plant-base oils, which are packed with nutrients that keep your skin looking youthful. They also help your digestion, and are full of antioxidants and beneficial compounds to help with long-term health. MUFAs are satisfying—they fill you up fast and for longer than many other foods. The top four MUFA-rich foods are:

- Vegetable oils, such as olive, canola, flaxseed, and safflower.
- Nuts and seeds (not peanuts).
- Olives.
- Avocados.

✳ TIP BOX

STORING OLIVE OIL
Researchers in Italy have found that light and heat destroys many of the disease-fighting compounds in olive oil. So store your oil in a dark, cool place and use within a month.

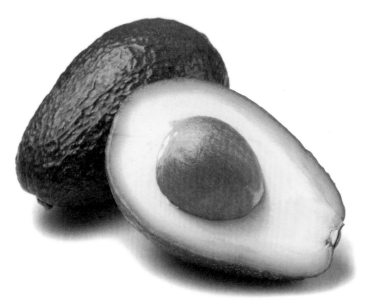

RIGHT As well as being a rich source of MUFAs, avocados are packed with nutrients, including antioxidant plant chemicals that can help lower blood cholesterol.

USING OIL

Aim to consume a couple of tablespoons of MUFA-rich oil a day. Oils vary greatly in quality, so buy the best that you can afford. Early pressings of oils such as olive and flaxseed are richer in beneficial plant chemicals, so choose extra-virgin oil that is cold-pressed. Extra-virgin olive is great for drizzling on salads and vegetables, and over prepared dishes, such as pasta or broiled meats. Flaxseed or hemp oils can be used in the same way, or you can add a spoonful to boost the nutrients in your morning smoothie.

For cooking, seek out canola oil. It is almost as rich a source of MUFAs as olive oil, and is particularly high in omega-3 fats.

USING NUTS AND SEEDS

Buy unshelled nuts because they will be fresher when you eat them. If you are buying shelled for convenience, be sure to choose the natural, salt-free type. Store in an airtight container and keep in a dark, cool place.

Nuts are perfect snack foods, and they are great additions to salads and stir-fries. Seeds are another good snack item, and can be sprinkled on salads and cereals.

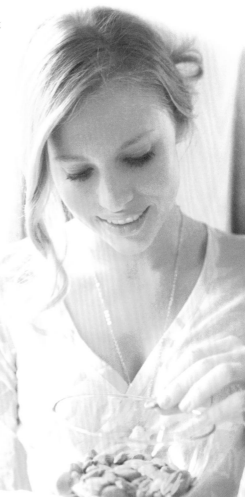

BELOW Eating a couple of servings of nuts—such as almonds or walnuts—each day can help you to feel full and maintain a stable weight.

☞ MAKE YOUR OWN...

NUT BUTTERS

Nut butters are easy to make, taste a whole lot better than store-bought types and are totally free of preservatives, salt, and sugar. Simply process shelled, roasted nuts in a food processor with a spoonful of olive oil—and use as a spread. They are great on plain bread or toast or you can pep up bland foods by spreading a little nut butter over them. Store in the refrigerator and use within a month.

06

Eat more fish

Fish is the most abundant form of food on the planet, largely due to the fact that so much of the earth is covered by the oceans. Apart from offering tremendous choice and variety, fish is remarkably good for you. It is unquestionably one of the best anti-aging food sources.

WHY IS FISH SO GOOD FOR YOU?

All types of fish and shellfish are a great source of protein, vitamins, and minerals. The United States Department of Agriculture (USDA) advises that we eat at least two portions a week. One of these should be oily fish.

OMEGA-3 FATTY ACIDS

Studies have shown that a diet that is rich in long-chain omega-3 fatty acids may help to improve a person's ability to concentrate and reduce the risk of the onset of dementia and Alzheimer's disease. Omega-3 fats also have an anti-inflammatory effect that may help relieve the symptoms of rheumatoid arthritis as well as skin problems, such as psoriasis. Additionally, and key to helping you stay young, omega-3 fats may help keep the heart healthy by making the blood less likely to clot, lowering blood pressure, and encouraging the muscles lining the artery walls to relax, improving the flow of blood to the heart.

Although omega-3 fats are also found in plant sources, the long-chain omega-3s found in oil-rich fish are the most beneficial kind for the body.

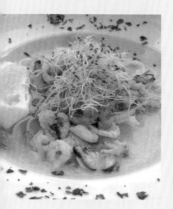

ABOVE Fish is an incredibly varied and adaptable food source. It can be used to make all kinds of dishes—like this shellfish soup—and it's all good for you, too!

RIGHT Oily fish, such as this mackerel, are high in omega-3 fatty acids and are particularly effective at preventing the ravages of time on both the heart and the brain.

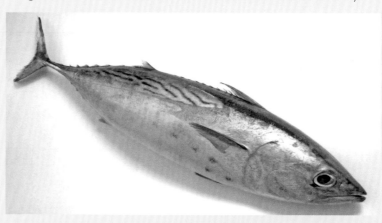

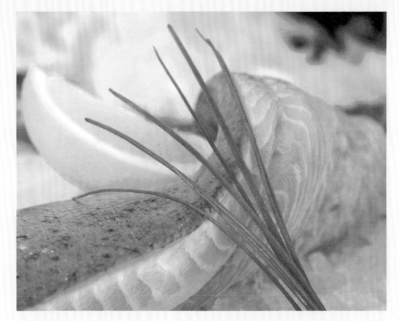

RIGHT Fish and seafood, in general, come in lots of different colors and textures. All types offer health benefits, but it is worth acquainting yourself with the particular properties of each species.

OTHER BENEFITS OF FISH

Oil-rich fish are one of the few foods that contain vitamin D, which is essential for calcium absorption. They also provide iodine and selenium, which are important trace elements that benefit the body and help maintain its youthfulness.

White fish are particularly low in fat—whichever species you choose. For example, 3½ ounces of haddock contains less than one per cent of fat. Being lower in fat also means that white fish are lower in calories, which makes them good for your waistline as well as your general health. The texture of white fish is also light and delicate, making the flesh easy to digest.

Although some shellfish contain high levels of cholesterol, this is not responsible for raised levels in the blood. The cause is a diet high in saturated fats that the body itself then turns into cholesterol in the blood.

☞ MAKE YOUR OWN...

FISH PASTE

It is very easy to make your own delicious fish paste. Select white fish with very firm meat—pollock or cod are particularly good. Crush the fish into a smooth paste using a traditional mortar and pestle, or use a blender. Wait until the fish has completely disintegrated, and then add egg white, starch, and seasoning. All the ingredients should be kept at a very cold temperature. You can use an ice cube during blending to keep the temperature low.

07

Reduce saturated fats & sugar

In order to stay healthy and feeling young, you need at least some fat and sugar in your diet. However, it is important to understand which are the beneficial kinds of fat and sugar and to make efforts to reduce your consumption of those that will damage your health.

WHAT ARE THE DIFFERENT KINDS OF FAT?

There are two main types of fat:

- Saturated fat ("bad" fat), which is largely derived from animal and dairy products. Having too much of this kind of fat can increase the amount of cholesterol in the blood, which increases the chance of developing heart disease. This is why it is important to reduce the amount of saturated fat that you consume by following the advice on these pages.

- Unsaturated fat ("good" fat), which comes in vegetable oils and various other forms. Consuming unsaturated fat instead of saturated fat will lower blood cholesterol and generally improve your health. Try to cut down on food that is high in saturated fat and instead have foods that are rich in unsaturated fat, such as vegetable oils (including sunflower, canola, and olive oil), oily fish, avocados, nuts, and seeds.

FOODS HIGH IN SATURATED FAT

In order to cut the amount of saturated fat in your diet and reduce the likelihood of heart disease or a stroke, try to eat the following foods less often or in smaller amounts:

- Meat pies, sausages, and meat with visible white fat.
- Hard cheese.
- Butter and lard.
- Pastry.
- Cakes and cookies.
- Cream, sour cream, and crème fraîche.
- Coconut oil, coconut cream, or palm oil.

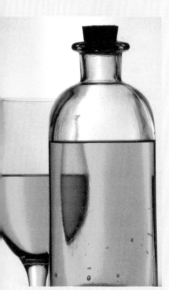

ABOVE There is really no need to cook using saturated animal fats when olive oil will give you just as tasty a result with no risk to your health.

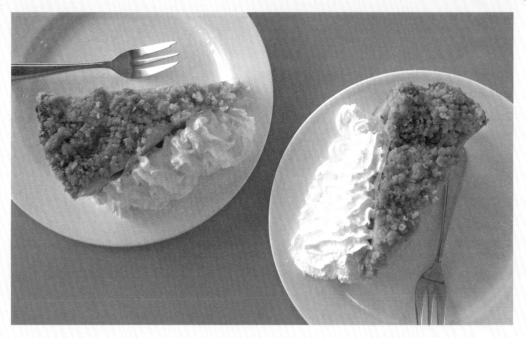

For a healthy choice, use just a small amount of vegetable oil or a reduced-fat spread instead of butter or lard. And when you are having meat, try to choose lean cuts and cut off any visible fat.

EAT LESS SUGAR

Many people eat far too much sugar than is good for them. We should all be trying to eat fewer foods containing added sugar, such as candies, cakes, and cookies, and drinking fewer sugary sodas and other soft drinks. Whatever age you are, it is in your interests to cut down on these kinds of foods. Your health will benefit very quickly as a result.

Consuming sugary foods and drinks too often can cause tooth decay, especially if you have them between meals. Additionally, many foods that contain added sugar are also high in calories, so cutting down on them could help you control your weight.

ABOVE Naughty... but nice—yet is it really worth it? Too much cake and cream will put inches on your waistline and years on your internal age.

08

Consume less salt

Many of us eat too much salt. This can lead to raised blood pressure, which puts you at an increased risk of health problems, such as heart disease and stroke. Cutting down on salt will keep you healthier and younger and it is not as hard as you might think.

HOW DO I CUT DOWN?

A few simple steps can help you to cut your salt intake:

- Read food labels thoroughly and buy products that contain less salt.
- Don't add salt when you are cooking.
- Put the salt shaker away—literally, don't put it on the table at meal times and then you won't add salt to your food.
- Use spices that do not contain sodium instead—for example, garlic, herbs, and pepper.
- Avoid prepared meals and canned and dried foods.

Remember that you don't have to add salt to food to be eating too much: 75 percent of the salt we eat is already in food when we buy it.

FOODS THAT CONTAIN SALT

Use food labels to help you cut down on salt:
- A high salt content is more than 1.5 gram salt per 100 gram (or 0.6 gram sodium).
- A low salt content is 0.3 gram salt or less per 100 gram (or 0.1 gram sodium).

Some foods are almost always high in salt because of the way they are made. Other foods, such as bread and breakfast cereals, can contribute a lot of salt to your diet. But that's not because these foods are always high in salt: it's because we eat a lot of them.

The following foods are almost always high in salt. To cut down on salt, eat them less often or have smaller amounts:
- anchovies
- bacon
- cheese
- gravy mixes

✳ TIP BOX

READ FOOD LABELS
These days the dangers of too much salt are widely appreciated, and this awareness is reflected in the detailed information labels on food packaging. Always check salt levels carefully before buying packaged foods, especially prepared meals.

- ham
- olives
- pickles
- salami
- salted and dry roasted nuts
- salt fish
- shrimp
- smoked meat and fish
- soy sauce
- bouillon cubes
- yeast extract

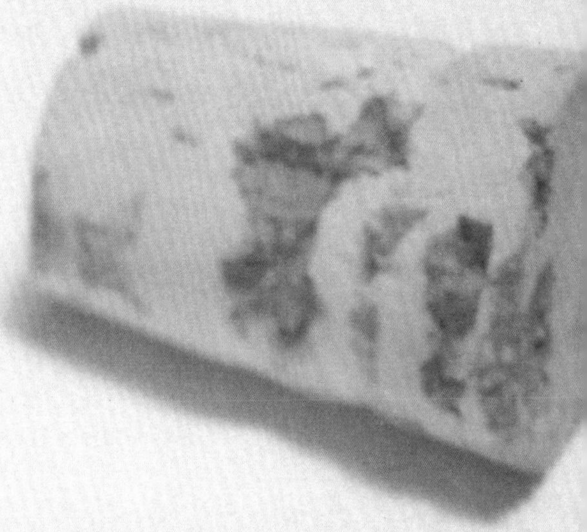

FOODS THAT CAN BE HIGH IN SALT

In these foods, the salt content can vary widely between different brands or varieties. That means you can cut down on salt by comparing brands, and choosing the one that is lower in salt. Food labels can help you do this.

These foods include:
- bread products, such as bagels and ciabatta
- pasta sauces
- potato chips
- pizza
- prepared meals
- soup
- sandwiches
- sausages
- ketchup, mayonnaise, and other condiments
- breakfast cereals

Adults should eat no more than 6 grams of salt a day: that's around one teaspoon. As a rule, aim for foods that have a low or medium salt content. Leave salty foods for only occasional consumption.

SALT AND SODIUM

Salt is also called sodium chloride. Sometimes food labels may list salt as sodium. However, there is a simple way to work out how much salt you are eating from the sodium figure:

- Salt = sodium x 2.5

Balance your weight

Nowadays there is a lot of discussion about the different components of food and the best ways to combine and balance them all together. However, the most important thing to remember is that whether you are consuming carbohydrates, fats, or proteins, all of them contain calories.

THE CALORIC BALANCE EQUATION

When it comes to maintaining a healthy weight, the bottom line is that calories count—in whatever form they come. A calorie is defined as a unit of energy supplied by food, and caloric balance is like a scale. Successful weight management is all about balance—balancing the number of calories that you consume with the number of calories that your body uses or "burns off" in the course of the day, through normal body functions, daily activities, and exercise.

MAINTAINING YOUR WEIGHT

We all have an optimum weight, which can be accurately assessed by checking your Body Mass Index (BMI). This is a measure of body fat based on height and weight that applies to adult men and women. A normal BMI reading is considered to be between 18.5 and 24.9. If your caloric balance is sound and you are eating roughly the same number of calories that your body is using, your weight and, therefore, your BMI will remain stable. In terms of balancing your weight, this is the ideal goal throughout your adult life.

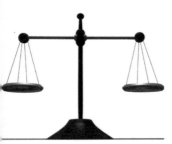

ABOVE So much of life—and about staying young and making the most of it—is about balance. Your weight is no exception.

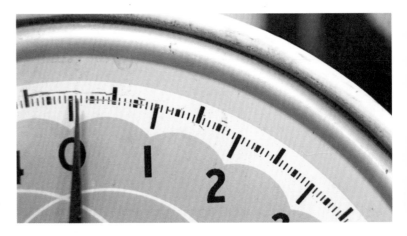

RIGHT Monitor your weight, BMI, and calorie intake on a regular basis and make changes to your diet as necessary.

GAINING WEIGHT

If you put on weight, you are in "caloric excess" instead of caloric balance, which means that you are eating more calories than your body is using. If this is the case, you will store these extra calories as fat and you will inevitably gain weight over a period of time. This will increase your BMI (a reading over 25 is deemed "overweight" and anything over 30 denotes obesity), which will put your heart under greater stress and could result in a wide range of health problems.

LOSING WEIGHT

In our fat-obsessed society, many people forget that being underweight can be just as dangerous as being overweight. If you are underweight, the chances are that you are in "caloric deficit." This means that you are eating fewer calories than you are using. Your body is pulling from its fat storage cells for energy, so your weight is decreasing.

AM I IN CALORIC BALANCE?

If you are maintaining your current body weight, you are in caloric balance. However, if you need to gain weight or to lose weight, you will need to tip the balance scale in one direction or another to achieve your goal. If you need to tip the balance scale in the direction of losing weight, bear in mind that it takes approximately 3,500 calories below your caloric needs to lose a pound of body fat. This means that to lose about one to two pounds per week, you will need to reduce your caloric intake by 500–1,000 calories per day.

To discover how many calories you are currently eating, begin writing down the foods you eat and the beverages you drink each day. By writing down what you eat and drink, you will become more aware of everything that you are putting into your mouth and this should help you to balance your weight more easily. By the same token, keep a record of the physical activity that you do and match this regularly against your caloric intake.

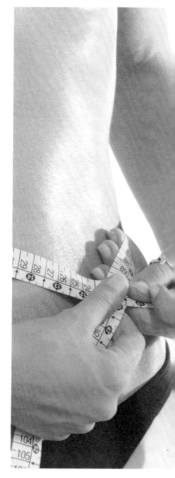

ABOVE The tape measure never lies. Consistently balancing your weight will keep you healthier and feeling younger.

CALORIE COUNTING

A simple guide to calorie counting is:

• **You need 2,361 calories per day to maintain your weight.**

• **You need 1,861 calories per day to lose 1 pound per week.**

• **You need 2,861 calories per day to gain 1 pound per week.**

10

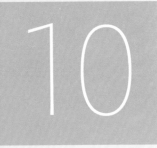

Eat three superfoods per day

Superfoods are rich in phytochemicals that can ward off such modern-day ills as heart disease, cancer, and osteoporosis. Eat these powerful foods often for incredible health and fitness benefits and to keep you looking and feeling as young as possible. Here are the top ten.

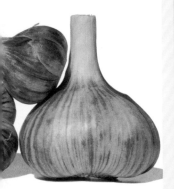

ABOVE If you don't already cook regularly with garlic, now might be a good time to start. Few foods will do your health more good than this incredibly versatile bulb.

TOP TEN SUPERFOODS

1 SOY Soy products contain all the amino acids required to create a complete protein, making them ideal substitutes for meat and fish.

2 LEAFY GREENS Dark green leafy vegetables, such as broccoli or collard greens, are a rich source of the nutrients that suppress the growth of cancer cells.

3 GARLIC Along with its cousins the shallot, onion, and leek, garlic has many benefits. It boosts immune function and regulates cholesterol and blood pressure levels to prevent heart disease and stroke.

4 WHEATGRASS JUICE As a potent detoxifier and antibacterial agent, wheatgrass clears poisons from the body and enhances immune and liver function.

5 SHIITAKE MUSHROOM Mushrooms are valued as powerful cancer fighters. They help fight disease by stimulating the immune system.

6 FLAXSEED OIL This is a beneficial omega-3 essential fatty acid (EFA)—essential for optimal brain and cell function, but also the building block for the hormones that regulate your body's inflammation systems.

7 GREEN TEA Low on caffeine and high on catechins, green tea is one of the best antitumor foods. Studies have shown that drinking green tea daily for at least six months reduces the chances of contracting cancer.

8 SEAWEED This family of sea vegetables is extremely high in antioxidants, fiber, magnesium, potassium, and iron. Seaweed also contains many anti-inflammatory, immune-boosting, and tumor-suppressing constituents.

9 BLUEBERRIES Although we usually think of citrus fruits as the main source of vitamin C, blueberries are an excellent source of this vital nutrient.

10 ALMONDS These tasty nuts have tremendous health potential. They are high in fat—but it's the "good" fat. They are also packed with vitamins and minerals.

Take essential vitamins

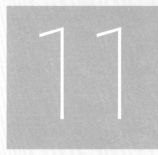

Vitamins are essential substances that cannot be manufactured by the body. We all need small amounts of vitamins for growth and development and in order to stay healthy and live a long life. Without vitamins the body simply cannot survive. Take them daily as supplements to your diet.

WHAT ARE VITAMINS?

The term vitamin is derived from the phrase "vital amine." There are two types.

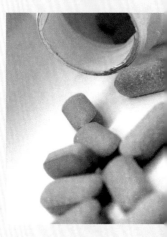

• **Fat-soluble vitamins (A, D, E, and K)** are usually found in meat and meat products, animal fat, and vegetable oils, dairy products, and fish. They are transported around the body in fat, and your body stores any excess in the liver and fatty tissues. This means that you do not need to get them from food sources every day.

• **Water-soluble vitamins (B, C, folic acid)** are found in meat, fish, fruit, vegetables, and whole grains. They are transported around the body in water. This means your body cannot store them because you pass the excess through urine. You need to eat foods containing these vitamins every day. Water-soluble vitamins can be destroyed by cooking, so steam and broil foods instead of boiling them.

MAKING SURE YOU GET WHAT YOU NEED

We all need vitamins to live a long and healthy life, and a varied diet is essential if we are to obtain the nutrients we need. Plenty of foods naturally contain vitamins, and some popular foods, such as breakfast cereals, are fortified with vitamins and minerals. If for any reason you are unable to get all the vitamins that you need from your daily diet—perhaps due to having a chronic illness—then it is important to supplement your meals with vitamin pills and liquids that are widely available from health stores and supermarkets.

ABOVE Vitamins will benefit your health, but it is important to take the right types in the correct amounts. Read labels thoroughly and consult a professional if in doubt.

DON'T TAKE TOO MANY!

Too little of just one vitamin may disturb your body's balance and cause health problems, but taking too many vitamins can also be dangerous. This is especially true of the fat-soluble vitamins A, D, E, and K, because it is harder for the body to get rid of any excess through urine.

37

12

Cook in a healthier way

When you are trying to adopt healthy eating habits and stay as young as you can for as long as you can, how you cook your food is just as important as what you eat. It is possible to prepare your favorite recipes using basic cooking methods that use less fat than traditional approaches.

Even making minor changes to your cooking methods will go a long way to help you achieve your weight management and health goals. The healthy cooking methods described below are a better option than eating fried food, and retain nutrients in a far more effective way, as well as the flavor of the foods.

STEAMING
Light steaming is one of the healthiest cooking methods, and is particularly well suited to cooking vegetables. Steaming retains the nutrients of food very well, and is an easy technique to master. Simply place the food in a perforated basket and suspend it above simmering water. You can add seasonings to the water to flavor the food as it cooks.

STIR-FRYING
Stir-frying is a healthy cooking method because it only requires a little vegetable oil, as opposed to the saturated fats associated with traditional frying methods. Because stir-fried vegetables are cooked for a very short period, they retain more of their nutrients as well as their texture, flavor, and color. However, one thing to bear in mind when stir-frying is that when oils are heated to a very high temperature, they become oxidized and release unhealthy free radicals. For this reason, a better way to stir-fry is to first add a little water to the skillet, then add a little oil, followed by a seasoning, such as ginger.

BROILING
Broiling food, or grilling it over a barbeque, is another cooking technique that is good for preparing low-fat, healthy meals. However, be careful to avoid charring the meat because this has been linked to an increased risk of some cancers. Trim excess fat and limit the amount of oil you add. Marinate meats before grilling and let the fat drip away from the food as it cooks.

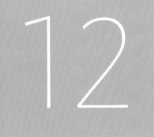

ABOVE Steamed vegetables taste delicious and are very good for you, as steaming is the best cooking method for retaining flavor and wholesomeness.

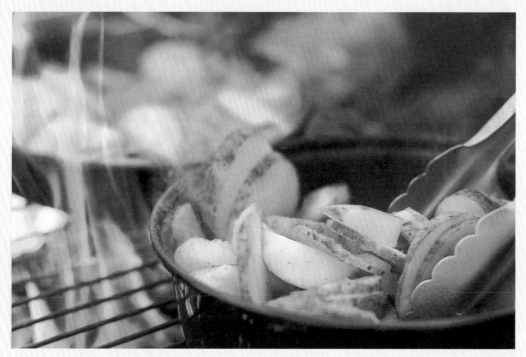

ROASTING AND BAKING

Roasting is similar to baking food, but is usually done at higher temperatures. Roasting is good for meat, poultry, seafood, and vegetables. To keep your roast as healthy as possible, lightly coat the food with olive oil and put a rack in the roasting pan so that the fat can drip away from the food. Additionally, use fat-free liquids, such as lemon juice, to baste the food in place of the pan drippings. Roasted vegetables are a delicious way to include more vegetables in your diet, but remember to roast the vegetables in a separate pan if you are having them with meat, so that the fat from the meat does not end up soaked into the vegetables.

POACHING

Poaching involves gently simmering food in water or a flavorful liquid until it is cooked through. It is important to remember to not let the liquid boil. It is a healthy method of cooking foods that are naturally tender such as eggs, fruits, chicken, and fish. Try poached eggs for a healthy and instant way of adding protein to a meal.

ABOVE Grilling or broiling works for many different kinds of food, but it's important not to let the meat char and to drain any excess fat away before serving.

13

Balance your diet

A diet based on starchy foods, such as rice and pasta, with plenty of fruit and vegetables, some protein-rich foods, such as meat, fish, and lentils, and some milk and dairy foods (as well as not too much fat, salt, or sugar) will give you all the nutrients that you need to stay young longer.

BALANCE FOR GOOD HEALTH

When it comes to a healthy diet, balance is the key to getting it right. This means eating a wide variety of foods in the right proportions. However, in our hectic modern lives, achieving that balance can sometimes be difficult. At the end of a long day, it can be tempting to grab the first prepared meal that comes to hand on the supermarket shelf. It is fine to do this occasionally, but many prepared meals contain high levels of fat, added sugar, and salt. If you consume prepared meals too often, at the expense of fresh whole foods, they will upset the balance in your diet.

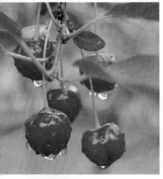

THE FIVE KEY FOOD GROUPS

All the food we eat can be divided into five groups. For a healthy diet, you need to eat the right balance of these groups:
- Fruit and vegetables.
- Starchy foods, such as rice, pasta, bread, and potatoes. Choose whole-grain types whenever you can.
- Meat, fish, eggs, and beans.
- Milk and dairy foods.
- Foods containing fat and sugar.

Many people eat too much fat, sugar, and salt, and not enough fruit, vegetables, and fiber.

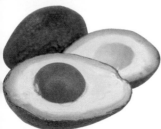

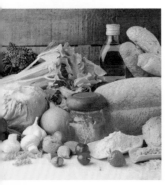

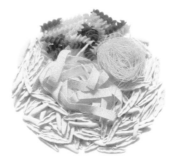

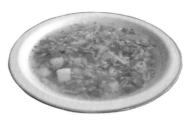

FIBER FROM FRUIT AND VEGETABLES

Fruit and vegetables are a vital source of vitamins and minerals. Ideally, you should eat at least five portions of a variety of fruit and vegetables every day. There is evidence that people who eat at least five portions a day are at lower risk of heart disease, stroke, and some cancers.

ENERGY FROM STARCH

Starchy foods, such as bread, cereals, potatoes, pasta, and corn are an important part of a healthy diet. They are a good source of energy and the main source of a range of nutrients in our diet. Starchy foods are fuel for your body. Starchy foods should make up around one-third of everything you eat.

PROTEIN FROM MEAT, FISH, EGGS, AND BEANS

These foods are all good sources of protein, which is essential for growth and repair of the body. They are also good sources of a range of vitamins and minerals. Around 15 percent of the calories that we eat each day should come from protein.

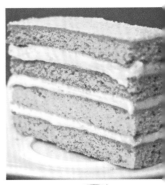

MILK AND DAIRY FOODS FOR CALCIUM AND PROTEIN

Cheese and yogurt are good sources of protein. They also contain calcium, which helps to keep your bones healthy and strong. However, some dairy products are high in saturated fat, which can raise blood cholesterol levels and increase the risk of heart disease.

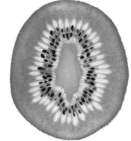

FAT AND SUGAR IN MODERATION

Many people eat too much fat and too much sugar, and this is one of the fastest ways to accelerate the aging process. Fats and sugar are both good sources of energy for the body, but if you eat too much of them, you will consume more energy than you burn. This generally means that you will put on weight. This can lead to obesity, which will increase your risk of type 2 diabetes, heart disease, and certain cancers.

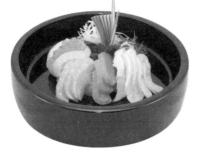

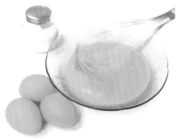

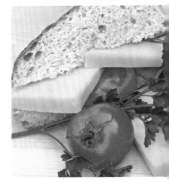

14

Eat to beat high blood pressure

High blood pressure is bad news for your health. If left unchecked, it can lead to a stroke or heart attack as well as damage to the kidneys and eyes. The good news is that you can do things with your diet to keep your blood pressure low or to bring it down if it is already high.

DO I HAVE HIGH BLOOD PRESSURE?

The big problem with high blood pressure is that most people who have it don't have any symptoms and so are not aware of their condition. Whether your doctor has told you that you have it or not, following these healthy eating tips should help you keep your blood pressure under control.

LOSE WEIGHT

The first thing you can do to help your blood pressure is to eat less and lose weight. These days many of us simply consume too many calories every day, which leads to an increased waistline and greater pressure on the heart and other organs. However, cut back on calories and do more exercise and you should find that your weight and blood pressure will soon drop.

CUT DOWN ON SALT

If you are at risk of high blood pressure, it is also very important to reduce your sodium intake (from salt). Sodium attracts water like a sponge, which can increase blood volume and blood pressure. It has been estimated that reducing sodium by one-third can reduce the incidence of strokes by as much as 22 percent and heart attacks by 15 percent. Professional recommendations are that adults should not consume more than 2.5 grams of sodium every day, which amounts to 6.25 grams of salt. The only real way to meet these targets is to cut down on processed foods and scrutinize food labels. As a rule of thumb, 0.5 grams sodium or more in a main meal (or per 3½ ounces/100 grams of snack food) is a high amount.

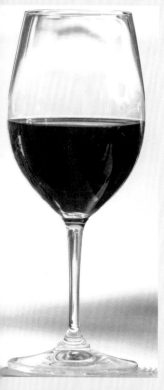

ABOVE A little red wine taken on a regular basis will actually help keep your blood pressure down, but too much will have the opposite effect.

REDUCE YOUR ALCOHOL INTAKE

Another factor to consider is alcohol. Alcohol constricts blood vessels, thus increasing blood pressure, and avoiding it leads to a prompt fall in blood pressure. U.S. government guidelines on alcohol are that men should not exceed two drinks daily and women one drink. (One drink is 5 ounces of wine, 1½ ounces of distilled spirits, or 12 ounces of regular beer.)

EAT MORE FRUIT, VEGETABLES & WHOLE GRAINS

Yes, you guessed it—when it comes to reducing blood pressure, once again our old friends fruit and vegetables can help. Eating lots of fruit, vegetables, and whole grains means you will increase your potassium levels—and it is a high potassium to sodium ratio that is most critical to lowering blood pressure, not just low sodium alone.

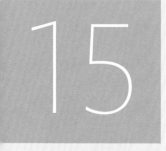

15

Eat mindfully

How often do you really think about what you eat and the way that you eat it? Are you really aware of just how much you eat and of what? Like anything else, you can educate the way that you eat and glean health benefits and aids to sustained youthfulness in the process. It's known in the dieting world as "eating mindfully."

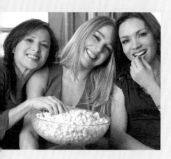

ABOVE Eating without any thought for your health can be fun, but is not such a good idea all the time. Eat mindfully and stay young!

MINDLESS EATING

Mindless eating. We all do it. Eating without really even being aware of how much we are eating. Here's an example: You are going to see a movie at the theater with a friend. After buying your tickets, you stop in the foyer and lick your lips over the popcorn, sodas, and hot dogs available. Before you know it, you've bought a king-size bucket of popcorn. After all, what's the point of going to the movie theater without popcorn? And the king-size bucket is better value, right? Next, you become so engrossed in the movie that, before it's even finished, you and your friend have eaten the whole bucket, right down to the very last kernel! Without a second's thought. That is mindless eating.

BECOMING MINDFUL

So how can you stop consuming extra—and almost certainly unnecessary and possibly unwanted—calories in this way? How can you become more in tune with the sensation of fullness in your stomach, of learning how to stop when you've had enough? By learning how to eat mindfully.

Becoming aware of what you are eating, or eating mindfully, takes some practice. You begin to pay more attention to what you are eating. You also begin to pay attention to those things that influence you to eat more—not only the external factors, but those that come from within, as well.

EATING MINDFULLY

If you want to eat mindfully, you should:
- Take the time to chew your food thoroughly—at least 20 times for each mouthful.
- Put down your utensils between bites, making an effort to stop several times during eating to check in with your stomach.
- Be aware of how you are feeling as you eat.

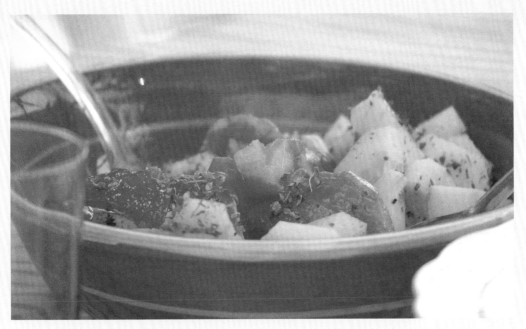

By becoming in touch with yourself in this way, you will gain the power to decide whether to continue eating because you are still genuinely hungry, or to say "enough" and to push your chair away from the table. Having this kind of control over your eating means that it is no longer a matter of how much food is left on your plate and whether you finish the plateful for the sake of it. Instead, it is about managing your enjoyment of one of the great pleasures in life without stuffing yourself and eating gratuitously.

Mindful eating is meant to bring enjoyment back to what you eat, thinking of your eating moment by moment. Remember:
• Slow down
• Become aware
• Eat as if this is the only food you will get all day
• Stop when you are full.

Mindful eating takes practice because of the possible disconnect between your mind and stomach. This is a disconnect that may have been going on for so long, you can no longer tell when you are full! However, do persist with this useful mind-over-matter technique; you will enjoy your food more and your waistline will surely benefit in the long run.

ABOVE Think about the content of the meals you prepare and then be aware of yourself and how you feel as you eat them. This is mindful eating.

45

Drink fruit smoothies

One great way to get some of your "five a day" fruit and vegetables is to make and drink fruit smoothies. There are numerous recipes available and you can also experiment and create new blends to your heart's content. Here we offer a few tips and one completely irresistible smoothie recipe!

THE BEAUTY OF SMOOTHIES

A fruit smoothie is a blend of fruit—the whole fruit and nothing but the fruit. No additives, no preservatives—just a single fruit, or a combination of pretty much any fruits you desire. The fruits that you use in your smoothie will have a massive impact on the flavor of your drink and its quality as well. Remember, the drink that comes out of your juicer or blender will only be as good as the ingredients that you put in. Try to shop with this in mind. If you are making a healthy smoothie, it makes sense to avoid produce that is likely to have been sprayed with pesticides. If you are going to take the time and trouble to make your own drink, make it as good quality as it can possibly be, because this will benefit you in many different ways.

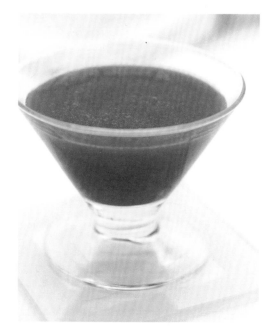

HEALTH BENEFITS OF SMOOTHIES

Fresh fruit juices and smoothies are abundant in enzymes responsible for the digestion and absorption of food into the body, ensuring optimal metabolism and high energy levels. Cooking fruit and vegetables destroys these enzymes, whereas juicing and blending releases them and lets the body utilize them easily. Another important health benefit is that juices and smoothies are generally low in fat and many of them are completely fat free.

Much of the way you look—and how old you look—is dictated from within your body, so it is as important to cleanse the inside of your body as it is the outside. Many of the nutrients found in fresh fruit smoothies help to rid the body of toxins, which in turn leads to cleaner, brighter skin and fewer pimples. Regular consumption of these drinks will give you a positive glow.

STRAWBERRY AND PEACH SMOOTHIE

Try to use plain yogurt with live cultures when making this smoothie, because it contains beneficial bacteria that are good for the digestive system. If peaches are out of season, you could try bananas instead.

1 peach
1 cup strawberries
1 cup plain yogurt with live cultures

Preparation time 5 minutes Serves 1

Peel and pit the peach, then coarsely chop. Hull the strawberries and halve them if they are large. Put the fruit into a blender with the yogurt and blend until smooth and creamy. Serve immediately.

One serving contains:
Energy Cal 269.04
Protein g 12.53
Carbohydrate g 35.6
Sugars g 29.94 Fat g 7.93
Saturates g 1.97
Fiber g 3.91
Sodium g 1.56

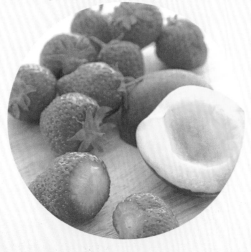

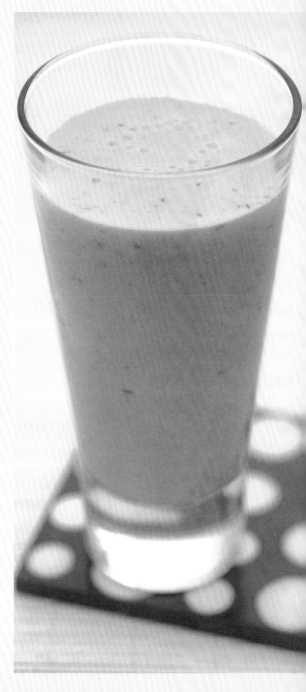

17

Avoid these foods

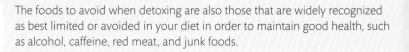

In order to stay as youthful and fit as possible, there are certain foods that should be largely avoided. Not only will the avoidance of these foods improve your health, it will also mean that you detoxify your entire system in the process, which is always beneficial.

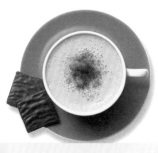

The foods to avoid when detoxing are also those that are widely recognized as best limited or avoided in your diet in order to maintain good health, such as alcohol, caffeine, red meat, and junk foods.

TEA, COFFEE, AND OTHER CAFFEINATED DRINKS

Caffeine is a diuretic and leads to dehydration. As a stimulant, it puts your body under stress and deprives it of essential nutrients. It also prevents your body from absorbing vitamins and minerals.

ALCOHOL

You should definitely give up alcohol while detoxifying. As well as containing sugar, alcohol is broken down into a toxin in your body, and the production of harmful free radicals is increased when it is being metabolized. Alcohol damages the liver, muscles, and brain, and depletes your body of essential vitamins and minerals.

BELOW Too many products made from wheat—bread, rolls, cereals, and so on—can have a negative effect on your general health and should be avoided.

WHEAT

Wheat bran can irritate the colon. Wheat protein (gluten) is difficult to digest, and may cause bloating, constipation, and/or diarrhea. Many people are intolerant of wheat but find they can consume other grains without problems. However, if you have celiac disease, you will need to avoid all sources of gluten permanently.

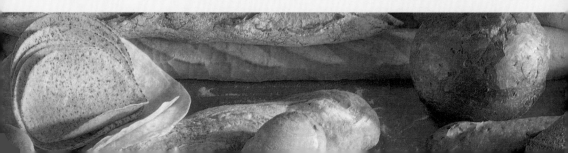

CONVENIENCE FOODS, FATTY AND/OR FRIED FOODS, AND PRODUCTS CONTAINING SUGAR

These include store-bought meals, cookies, cakes, and spreads. Soft drinks also contain sugar. Diet versions are not suitable alternatives because of the amount of additives they contain. Choose fresh or dried fruits and whole-food products instead, and drink water or fruit juices.

MEAT

Meat creates extra work for your digestive system and in the case of red meat contains a lot of harmful saturated fat. Eat small quantities of good-quality, organic protein instead to give your body the amino acids it needs. Eggs, oily fish (from unpolluted waters), and soy products are good choices.

SALT AND SUGAR

Your body needs a great deal of fluid to metabolize foods that are high in refined sugar, so if you eat a lot of these foods, your body will retain a lot of water as well. Sugar disrupts blood glucose (sugar) levels. Salt prevents fluid from being removed from the body.

COW'S MILK PRODUCTS

Milk increases the production of mucus in the body, so it is not beneficial when detoxing. In addition, many people lack sufficient quantities of the enzyme lactase, which is needed to digest lactose (the main sugar in milk) and, therefore, cannot properly digest dairy products.

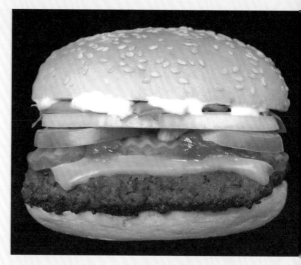

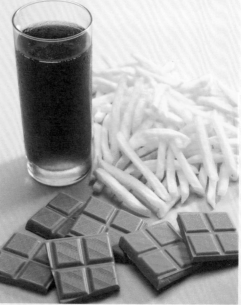

ABOVE Many people enjoy a burger now and again—and a multibillion dollar fast food industry testifies to that. However, they are best left alone.

49

Try a detox diet

Detoxing is good for you at any time in life, but as you get older it will be particularly beneficial and will help you feel younger. On the preceding pages, we looked at the foods you should avoid; however, there are lots of things that you can eat and drink that will positively aid the detoxification process.

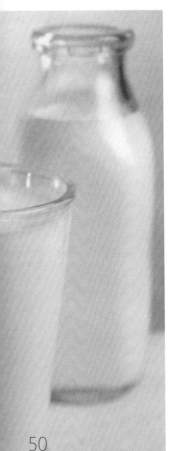

BELOW Alkaline probiotic drinks will help you detox quickly and effectively.

One of the key ways to detox is to keep the body in an alkaline state. The body's acid–alkaline balance adjusts throughout the day depending on the types of food we eat. Grains and proteins leave an acidic residue when metabolized; fruit and vegetables leave an alkaline residue. Protein and grains are essential for our overall health and well-being, but if you balance their intake with large amounts of fruit and vegetables your body is more likely to remain alkaline. Choose organic food and eat fruit and vegetables raw whenever possible to make sure you obtain the maximum amount of nutrients.

THE IMPORTANCE OF FLUIDS

Drinking plenty of fluids—at least six 8-fluid-ounce glasses a day—is essential for good health. It will help avoid fluid retention and keep your body's waste disposal system—the liver, kidneys, lungs, digestive system, lymphatic system, and skin—functioning efficiently. Water flushes out toxic materials, reduces bloating, helps keep your skin clear, and is essential for a successful detox.

Drink fluids throughout the day, reducing the intake in the hours leading up to bedtime so that you do not have to get up in the night. Drinking with meals dilutes the digestive enzymes, so try to avoid drinking just before or up to an hour after meals. Herbal teas are excellent alternatives to water, and green tea and Rooibosch tea are rich in antioxidants. Freshly squeezed fruit and vegetable juices are loaded with nutrients, antioxidants, and enzymes and help to keep your system alkaline, but they need to be drunk immediately because the nutrients are destroyed on exposure to air.

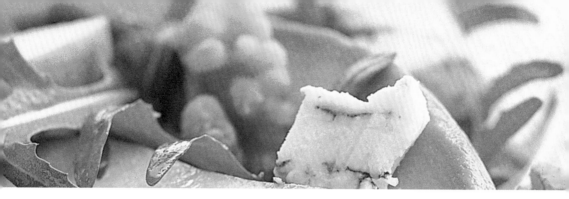

DETOX SUPERFOODS

Consume the following as often as you can.

APPLE Helps excrete heavy metals and cholesterol and is cleansing for the liver and kidneys.

ASPARAGUS Superb detox food because of its diuretic effect; helps maintain healing bacteria in the intestines.

BROCCOLI Like other members of the cabbage family, increases levels of glutathione, a key antioxidant that helps the liver expel toxins.

CARROT Packed with beta-carotene, a powerful antioxidant; antibacterial and antifungal.

CRANBERRY Antioxidant-rich; destroys harmful bacteria in the kidneys, bladder, and urinary tract.

FENNEL Has a strong diuretic action and helps the body eliminate fats.

GARLIC Powerful antioxidant that is also excellent at eliminating toxic microorganisms.

GINGER Relieves abdominal bloating, nausea, and diarrhea. Helps to stimulate digestive enzymes, aiding efficient digestion.

GLOBE ARTICHOKE Purifies and protects the liver and has a diuretic effect on the kidneys.

LEMON Stimulates the release of enzymes—an essential part of the liver's detoxification process.

OLIVE OIL Antioxidant; prevents cholesterol from being transformed into a harmful free radical.

ONION Rich in the antioxidant quercetin, which protects against free radical damage; onion enhances the activity of healthy intestinal flora and is antiviral.

PARSLEY Diuretic and helps kidneys to flush out toxins; contains phytonutrients that support the liver and is rich in antioxidants.

QUINOA Easily digested cleansing grain that is a good source of protein, vitamins, and minerals.

RICE Brown rice in particular cleans the intestines as it passes through and prevents constipation; anti-allergenic and helps stabilize blood-sugar levels.

SALAD GREENS Superb antioxidant and cleanser of the digestive tract.

SEAWEED Strong antioxidant; helps alkalinize the blood and strengthens the digestive tract.

TOMATO Rich source of the antioxidant lycopene, thought to prevent a variety of diseases.

WATERCRESS Purifies the blood and expels wastes from the body.

YOGURT Yogurt with live cultures contains probiotics that can reduce intestinal inflammation and fungal infections and eliminate bad bacteria that damage the intestinal wall.

19

Take detox supplements

Supplements are usually taken as a nutritional safeguard against possible vitamin and mineral deficiencies caused by modern diets. When you are detoxing, there are several supplements you can take that support the digestive processes and help nutrient absorption.

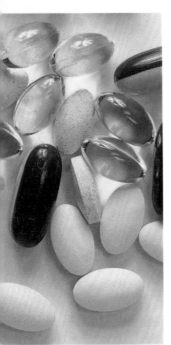

You shouldn't need to take a specific antioxidant supplement—if you are eating a variety of fruit and vegetables, you will be meeting your body's requirements. Too much vitamin C can cause diarrhea and stomach upsets, while excessive amounts of vitamin A can be toxic. A general multivitamin/multimineral supplement, however, is normally fine, though you should seek advice from a qualified person before taking any supplements.

Unless otherwise stated on the packaging, supplements should be taken after food and washed down with water. Some can cause indigestion or make you feel sick if eaten on an empty stomach.

BLUE-GREEN ALGAE
These are a rich source of over 100 easily assimilated nutrients, including antioxidants, vitamins, minerals, enzymes, essential fatty acids, amino acids, and proteins. A number of blue-green algae are widely available in supplement form, for example, aphanizomenon, chlorella, and spirulina. Dosage: 500–1500 mg twice a day, best taken with food.

CO-ENZYME Q10
This is a substance needed by enzymes to help in energy production. Co-enzyme Q10 is particularly active in the liver, where it helps in the breakdown of toxins. This powerful antioxidant also helps to keep the heart healthy. Dosage: 10–100 mg daily, best taken with food.

DANDELION
This increases the breakdown of dietary fats by stimulating the release of bile from the gallbladder. It is an extremely effective diuretic because of its high levels of potassium. Dosage: 500 mg twice a day.

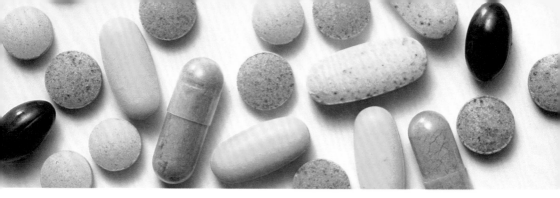

KELP

These supplements are derived from seaweeds and contain vitamins, amino acids, and minerals. Kelp is a particularly rich source of calcium, magnesium, potassium, iron, and iodine. Iodine improves production of thyroid hormones, which boost metabolic rate and may, therefore, help weight loss. Dosage: Depends on the supplement—take according to manufacturer's instructions. Note that some people are sensitive to iodine and taking kelp supplements can cause allergic reactions.

MILK THISTLE

The active compound in this antioxidant herb is silymarin, which helps repair the liver by encouraging the replacement of damaged liver cells with healthy ones. It also increases levels of glutathione, which helps remove alcohol, metals, and pesticides from the body. Dosage: 120–160 mg three times a day.

PSYLLIUM HUSKS

These husks contain insoluble fiber, which loosens old matter in the bowel and increases the bulk of stools, and soluble fiber, which absorbs toxins in the bowel. Dosage: 1,000–3,000 mg one to three times a day with at least two 8-fluid-ounce glasses of water. Not to be taken with food.

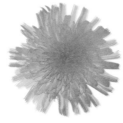

ABOVE Silymarin—commonly known as milk thistle—has been used for centuries as a purgative. It is particularly beneficial to the liver but, like all supplements, must be taken sparingly.

53

20

Improve your digestion

A quick and efficient digestive system is what's needed for optimal health and vitality. When the digestive system is slow and sluggish, the whole body is adversely affected. Problems with digestion can be obvious: belching, flatulence, bloating, or cramping. These symptoms can make you feel ill and old.

BELOW Avoid heavy cakes and rolls, which will clog your digestive system and make you feel bloated and sluggish. Instead, eat fresh fruit and vegetables and drink lots of water.

DRINK WATER ONLY BETWEEN MEALS

Water taken between meals aids digestion. It provides the necessary lubrication to keep the bowels moving smoothly, but ideally should be taken before and after meals instead of during them. An adequate intake of water aids the absorption of nutrients and the elimination of wastes by keeping the blood from getting too thick and becoming slow-moving. Ideally, drink eight to ten glasses of water per day, starting with two glasses upon rising. Drink another glass half an hour before each meal. Then drink another glass two hours after each meal.

AVOID OTHER DRINKS WITH MEALS

If you can manage it, don't drink anything with your meals. Drinking liquids while eating only dilutes digestive juices, making them less effective. This inhibits and slows the digestive process. However, sometimes it can feel difficult to swallow food properly without the assistance of a drink.

DON'T OVERDO FIBER

While elsewhere in this book we extol the virtues of fiber, it is possible to have too much of a good thing. Rough fiber, such as wheat bran, can actually damage the intestines by harshly scraping the mucus-lined membrane. If adequate water is not consumed, fiber can actually block the intestine.

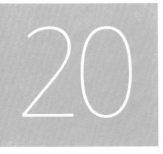

LEFT It is a recurring theme in this chapter, but fresh vegetables will always do you good and will help your digestion. Having said that, don't overdose on fiber.

RESTRICT THE VARIETY OF YOUR MEALS

Eat only a small variety of foods at each meal. While it is important to maintain a good balance of protein, carbohydrates, fats, and fiber, try to keep the mix relatively simple.

EAT IN A RELAXED ENVIRONMENT

If you find yourself feeling anxious during meal times, try to control the amount of stress that you experience while you are eating. It's often better to skip a meal when you are feeling stressed. Have a glass of water instead, until you are feeling calm.

CHEW FOOD PROPERLY

Digestion begins in the mouth. Take your time and chew.

☞ TRY THIS...

RECIPE FOR BETTER DIGESTION

This combination of roasted vegetables sprinkled with chives is a great traditional recipe for improving digestion.

FRENCH BRAISED CARROTS AND TURNIPS
You will need:
• 1 bunch carrots, cleaned
• 1 bunch turnips, peeled and halved
• 2 cups organic vegetable or chicken stock
• 2 tbsp honey or sugar
• 2 tbsp coconut oil or unsalted butter
• Chives, chopped (regular or garlic)
• Sea salt and fresh ground pepper to taste
To prepare:
• Cut carrots and turnips into ½-inch slices.
• Place the carrots and turnips in a large, heavy saucepan with the stock, sugar, or honey, coconut oil or butter, sea salt, and freshly ground organic pepper.
• Cook them, partially covered, over medium heat for about 20 minutes, until they are tender.
• Check the seasoning.
• Sprinkle with chopped chives and serve in a warmed serving dish.

55

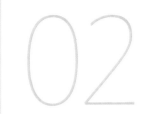

Fit mind, fit body

If you exercise regularly, you are sure to boost your self-esteem as well as your immune system and cardiovascular health. These benefits are key to staying young both inside and out. This chapter covers posture and breathing, and guides you through exercises to improve strength, energy, mobility, and flexibility. It also provides you with techniques for building exercise into your daily routine and for remaining motivated throughout your life.

Introduction

Exercise. You know you should do it, but sometimes it can be a struggle. However, if you can get yourself consistently into the right frame of mind, you will be amazed by how quickly you will be able to maintain a revivifying, invigorating regime that will keep you feeling young and healthy inside and out.

WHY EXERCISE?

If you are fortunate enough to enjoy basically good health, a largely consistent weight, and a body that you are relatively happy with, you might wonder just what is the point of exercise and why should you bother doing it? However, there are many compelling reasons to undertake a regular fitness program, particularly as you become older, no matter how well and content you might already feel. For starters, regular exercise will improve your mental health and general sense of well-being. As we say in the title of this chapter, fit mind, fit body—well, the principle also works the other way round. Secondarily, keeping your body toned and your mind honed will delay the inevitable aging process that befalls us all and will keep you feeling young and healthy for longer.

OTHER MAIN BENEFITS OF EXERCISE

There are all kinds of exercises covered in this chapter, designed to strengthen the core of your body, improve your posture, and stretch and tone all areas of your physique. We show you how to get into the right frame of mind for exercise, how to breathe properly while doing it, and how to make the most of its myriad positive effects. Although many of the exercises provided pertain to individual parts of the body, remember that you should aim for an holistic approach to your exercise that will benefit your entire being. The following general benefits will always accrue from any effective regular program:

- Regular exercise will help reduce your susceptibility to heart disease and stroke by improving blood flow, and increasing your heart's working capacity.
- Regular physical activity can reduce blood pressure in those with high blood pressure levels.
- Physical activity helps to reduce body fat by building or preserving muscle mass and improving the body's ability to use calories.
- By increasing muscle strength and endurance and improving flexibility and posture, regular exercise helps to prevent back pain.
- Studies on the psychological effects of exercise have found that regular physical activity can improve your mood and the way you feel about yourself.

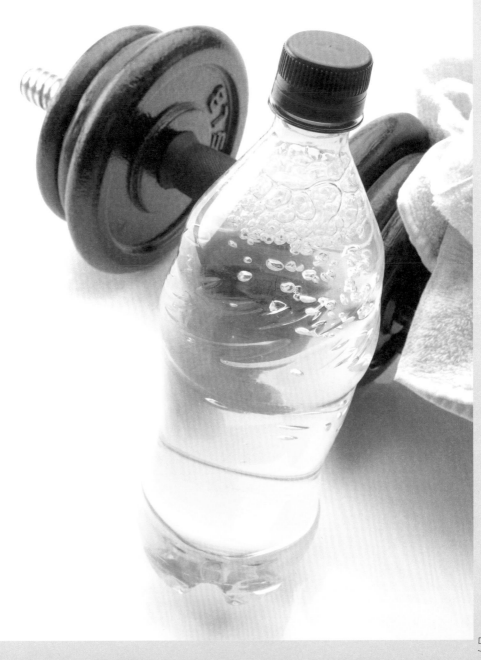

21

Breathe deeply and relax

Controlled breathing and simple muscle-relaxation techniques can be practiced to reduce the physical and mental effects of stress, which can cause a buildup of unwanted toxins in your body. If you find it difficult to begin a breathing and relaxation program on your own, try consulting a professional.

BREATHING

Breathing is essential for life: As you breathe, oxygen is taken into the lungs and released into the bloodstream, where it fuels the production of energy that enables your body to function. If you are stressed, your breathing tends to be shallow, using only the top part of the lungs. If you learn to breathe properly, you will benefit from a lower heart rate, reduced blood pressure, and lower levels of stress hormones.

HOW TO BREATHE DEEPLY

If you find your breathing is too fast or too shallow, the following exercise—known as abdominal breathing—will help you breathe more deeply. It uses the diaphragm, the sheet of muscle forming the top of the abdomen, to enable the lungs to inflate and deflate with minimal effort.

1 Sit in a comfortable position. Place one hand on your chest and the other over your diaphragm just below the breastbone. Breathe in slowly through your nose, and try to breathe so that the hand on your chest remains relatively still.

2 Hold the breath for a few seconds then breathe out slowly through your nose. Release as much air as possible.

3 Repeat three or four times.

LEFT Keep your eyes firmly closed and sit still as you prepare to concentrate hard on your breathing throughout the exercise.

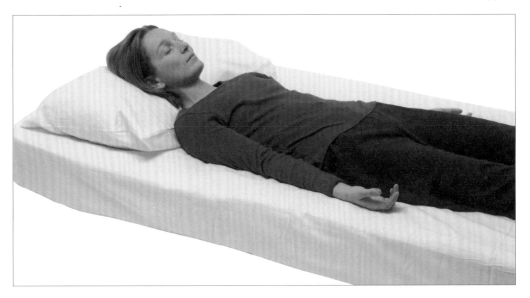

RELAXATION

When your body and mind are under pressure, your muscles become constricted. This restricts the blood supply, making it harder for the body to eliminate toxins, and can dramatically affect the way your body functions. The following technique will help you to relax all the major muscle groups.

1 Lie down with a pillow under your head for support. Close your eyes and focus on breathing slowly.

2 Tense the muscle in your right foot, hold for a few seconds, then release. Tense and release the calf, then the thigh muscles. Repeat with the left foot and leg.

3 Tense and release the muscles in your right hand and arm, then the left.

4 Tense and release each buttock, then the stomach muscles.

5 Lift your shoulders up to your ears, hold for a few seconds, then lower. Repeat three times. Rock your head gently from side to side.

ABOVE Lying down with your head comfortably supported by a pillow will immediately make you feel more relaxed.

BELOW Tense and release each of your muscles in turn. This shows the hand in a relaxed state.

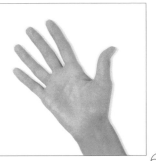

22

Achieve inner harmony

Meditation and visualization help you achieve and maintain inner harmony; they are also important for detoxing because they reduce stress levels. If stress persists, stress hormones interfere with the functioning of the circulatory and immune systems, making it harder for the body to detoxify properly.

If you are not used to meditating or visualization, you may find them hard to do at first, but regular practice will soon lead to their becoming second nature. As you become more experienced in controlling your mind, you may be able to switch to a relaxed state despite the distractions of the bustle of life around you.

KEY PRINCIPLES

A practitioner can show you how to achieve a meditative state, but you can teach yourself if you are sufficiently disciplined. In order to meditate successfully, there are a few basic requirements:

BELOW Meditation has been practiced for centuries in many different cultures as an effective way of relaxing both the mind and body.

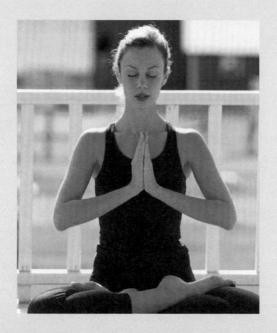

- A quiet place where you will not be disturbed. Ideally, this would be somewhere outside in the fresh air, where you can breathe freely and deeply and feel in touch with nature. Of course, if you live in a city, this could be tricky.

- Regular practice, preferably at the same time each day.

- An empty stomach.

- A comfortable position.

- A focus for the mind to help you withdraw from your surroundings.

BASIC MEDITATION

1 Sit up in a comfortable position with your spine straight. Keep your eyes open or closed, depending on the method of meditation you are using. Rest your hands in your lap.

2 Breathe slowly and rhythmically, and try to stay as still as possible.

3 Focus on the object of your meditation and allow your attention to be passive. If your mind starts to wander, acknowledge what is happening then return to your focus.

4 Continue for as long as is comfortable—for a few minutes to start with, building up to 20 minutes a day.

5 When you are ready, open your eyes, then take a minute to become fully aware of your surroundings.

VISUALIZATION

This is a technique that harnesses the imagination to create positive mental images to deal with stress and illness. Through imagination, you can use positive thinking to stimulate the body's natural healing abilities. Choose a quiet place where you won't be disturbed. Breathe slowly and relax. Focus on your chosen mental image. To combat stress, visualize a calm, beautiful scene and picture yourself there. Repeat positive affirmations as you do this.

23

Think yourself fit

If you struggle to maintain an exercise program or find it hard to keep those new year resolutions to stay fit, maybe the problem is in your mind rather than in your body. Sports psychologists are increasingly of the view that keeping fit is a state of mind as well as a physical objective.

MENTAL FITNESS FOR PHYSICAL FITNESS

Next time you are planning to go to the gym—or even just for a brisk walk—ask yourself why you exercise, what you are doing it for, what you hope to achieve. Be clear about your mental objectives, and your physical ones should become easier. Try the following steps to mental fitness:

- **What are your reasons for exercise?** Write them down one by one, in as much detail as possible. Then review them thoroughly and ask yourself if you are being completely honest about your motivation.

- **Set challenging but achievable goals.** Establish your ultimate goal, then work back to the present, putting in nearer-term, easier goals to achieve along the way. Put your goals into a timescale and have them in writing.

- **Learn to self-talk.** Everyone experiences times when they don't want to exercise, but those who go ahead and do it anyway are those who have learned to counter negative self-talk with positive, persuasive arguments.

- **When you are working out in the gym,** swimming in the pool, or going for a walk, try to stay "in the moment" throughout the experience, instead of switching off completely, or thinking about other things.

- **Mix things up and don't get stuck in a rut.** Have a sense of discovery and fun about exercise. Try a lot of different forms of exercise.

- **Use positive visualization** to help motivate you: picture yourself on the treadmill or taking part in that aerobics class before you actually exercise.

- **After your workout,** walk, swim, or whatever, take a moment to congratulate yourself—and reflect on what you've achieved.

✱ **TIP BOX**

TRY A PERSONAL TRAINER
If you are still having trouble motivating yourself in your exercise program after following these tips, consider using a personal trainer—they are widely available and often provide their services at surprisingly competitive rates.

OPPOSITE Change your approach to your exercise program by getting in touch with your mind and living "in the moment" before and as you workout.

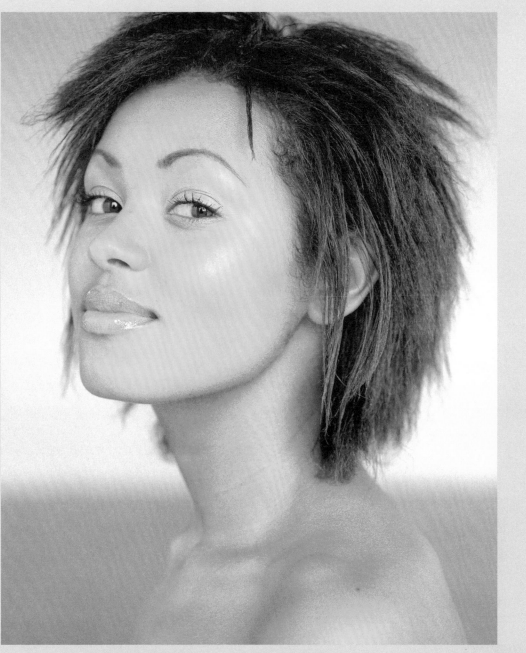

24

Stretch your mind

If you constantly do the same things over and over, your brain works on autodrive, simply following tried and tested automatic routines. Change things around and the brain has to create new cerebral pathways and build better networks. In a word, it has to work harder—which keeps it fit.

To keep your mind active, do something different—every day. You don't have to grapple with huge challenges; simply take a new route to work or buy a different newspaper.

Try using your nonwriting hand to brush your teeth or use your computer mouse, and move the things you reach for automatically in the morning, such as your alarm clock or your shower gel, to a different place. All these things will encourage your brain to wake up and force the lazy cell networks to work in new ways.

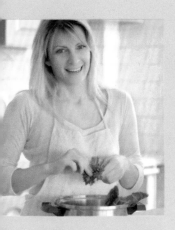

ABOVE Doing something as simple as trying an unusual recipe can give the brain something new to grapple with.

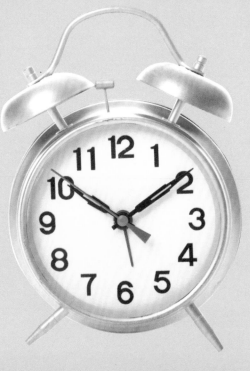

RIGHT Making minor changes to your routine, such as putting your alarm clock in a different place, can help stop the brain stagnating.

Stimulate your mind

Brain function naturally deteriorates from your mid-20s onward, but there is plenty that you can do to reverse the effects of time and keep the mind young and vital. The key thing is to keep yourself stimulated all the time with new and interesting learning experiences.

A simple daily activity, such as doing the crossword, can make all the difference to the way you think. Playing chess, or doing a cryptic crossword, challenges you to think laterally, and word games promote mental fluency. One research study found that people who did crosswords cut their risk of developing dementia by almost half.

- **Start a new hobby.** Doing any new activity helps to build new connections in the brain. Choose something that requires coordination between different parts of the brain such as tai chi, dancing, or learning a musical instrument.

- **Meditate.** Mindfulness practices, such as meditation, can improve memory and the ability to focus. One study at Massachusetts General Hospital found that over time, meditation thickened the cerebral cortex—the area of the brain associated with concentration and memory.

RIGHT As well as helping to manage stress, studies show that meditation can even affect the way the brain is wired, improving memory and concentration.

67

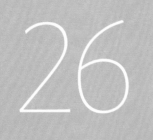

Get brain fit

As you get older, your brain will change, just like every other part of your body. In fact, it changes throughout your life. However, this isn't necessarily a bad thing—your brain might be aging, but it continues to respond and adapt to the environment you live in and the experiences that you have.

KEEPING YOUR BRAIN YOUNG

Scientists used to believe that we are born with a finite number of brain cells that begin dying off from the age of about seven years old. The theory was that this process causes an irreversible downward spiral in mental health and fitness. However, we now understand that this is not really the case. Brain cells are indeed lost in staggering numbers throughout life, but recent research has established that new ones are also created. You can maintain a healthy and vibrant brain throughout your life as long as you do what is necessary to keep new brain cells coming and then put them to proper use. Beyond making new brain cells, making more connections between those that you already have is also incredibly important. No matter if you are 10, 40, or 90 years old, the health of your brain is the single biggest factor that determines your quality of life.

THOUGHT CONTROL

Thoughts are electrical and chemical activities that by their very existence alter the physical structure of your brain. Although you can't stop the process, you can have some control over it. The brain is like any other "muscle" in your body. If you nourish it, exercise it, and rest it appropriately, it gets stronger. If you neglect to take care of it, you may lose brain function as it withers away. A combination of good diet, plenty of exercise, rest, and mental exercises, such as chess, su doku, or crosswords, will ensure that you are able to keep your thought control in prime condition.

THE THREE FOUNDATIONS OF BRAIN FITNESS

The fitness of your brain controls several kinds of intelligence. Each of these contributes to your success in different areas of your life, and each applies no matter what age you are:

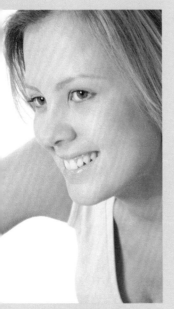

ABOVE Healthy mind, healthy body. The link between mental health and how you look and feel physically is undeniable.

- **Emotional intelligence (EQ)** is your ability to control your own emotions, regulate your mood, control your stress levels, and appropriately read the emotions of others. The more you work on your EQ, the more confident you will become.

- **Physical intelligence (PQ)** is your brain's ability to control your body. The brain controls your metabolism, body weight, immune system, heart rate, blood pressure, diet cravings, and nearly everything else. The higher your PQ, the smoother your body systems will function and the healthier you will be.

- **Cognitive intelligence (IQ)** is your intellect, creativity, and artistic talent. The higher your IQ, the greater your ability to remember what you have learned, solve problems, make decisions, and work creatively.

The important thing to appreciate is that all three of these areas of brain fitness are interlinked. In order to look after one area of your intelligence, you need to look after all the others.

RIGHT Emotional contentment is only one part of the mental fitness equation, but hugely important nonetheless.

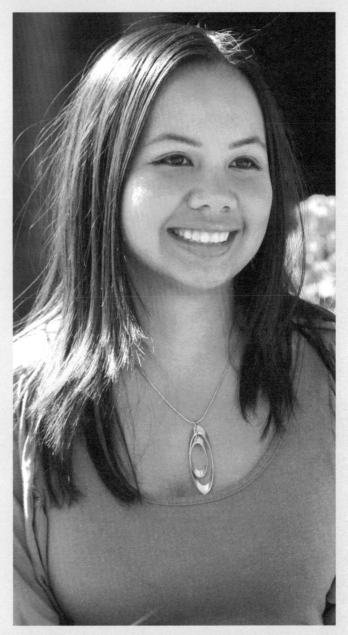

Strengthen your core

Core training is a workout that strengthens your body from the inside out by concentrating on the muscles that form your "core." The core of your body is simply what's between the shoulders and hips—basically, the trunk and pelvis. Core training reeducates these muscles to make them more effective.

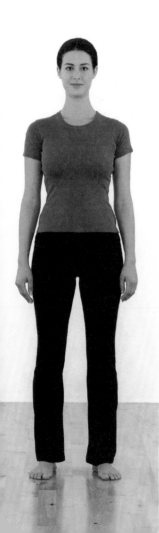

WHAT IS THE CORE?

The core is a crucial group of muscles, not only for sports throughout life, but for normal daily activities as well, because it comes into play just about every time you move. Draw an imaginary line around the center of your body, starting at your navel, and most of the muscles bordering that line are your core muscles.

The core acts to produce force (for example, during lifting), it stabilizes the body to permit other musculature to produce force (for example, during running), and it's also called upon to transfer energy (for example, during jumping). This is why it is so important that your core is strong. Once you have learned how to strengthen your core, your lower abdominal muscles will be drawn in toward the spine and help you sit up straight. Your balance and coordination will be improved, and, most important of all, the stability these muscles bring will help keep your spine healthy and flexible.

WHAT IS CORE STABILITY?

Core stability is the effective use of the core muscles to help stabilize the spine, allowing your limbs to move more freely. Good core stability means you can keep your midsection rigid without forces, such as gravity, affecting your movements. The positive effects of this include reducing the chance of injury, better posture, increased agility and flexibility, and improved coordination.

LEFT A strong core is the foundation of a healthy, youthful body.

HOW TO TRAIN YOUR CORE

Traditional abdominal training is not the ideal way to train your core. Endless crunches are not only monotonous, but also ineffective because they don't target the deep muscles. The abdominals are muscles just like any other and should be trained using the same principles as any other muscle group. This means they should be loaded with resistance, and challenged in a variety of ways—by lateral (side) flexion, bending forward and backward, and rotation. When starting out on a core training program, you need to progress properly:

- Start with the easiest movements and then move on to the more difficult ones.
- You may not require any extra load to start with but, as you adapt, you can increase the resistance, for example, by using weights or changing the position, etc.
- Perform all movements in a slow and controlled manner and gradually speed up.

- To increase the complexity and muscle demands of the exercises, many moves can be performed lying prone (face down) or supine (on your back) on an unstable platform after you have mastered them on the floor.

BELOW Training your core thoroughly on a regular basis will increase your energy levels and will pay dividends in greater fitness for years to come.

Improve your posture

The alignment of your muscles and joints is known as "posture." If your posture is consistently poor over a period of time, your muscles will be subjected to uneven stresses, leading to aching muscles and joints, tiredness, weakness, and an increased risk of injury when exercising.

GOOD POSTURE

Good posture looks natural and relaxed, not slouched and hunched. When you are standing up, your neck should be in line with your spine, with your head balanced squarely on top, your shoulder blades set back and down, and your spine long and curving naturally. Your hips should be straight.

HOW TO CHECK YOUR POSTURE

Stand sideways in front of a full-length mirror to assess your posture. Imagine there is a straight line drawn down the center of your body. If your posture is good, the line will pass through the center of the earlobe, the tip of the shoulder, halfway through the chest, slightly behind the hip, and just outside the ankle bone.

It does take time to correct any postural deficiencies you may have, but it is important to identify what your weaknesses are—for example, rounded shoulders—so that you can work on correcting these. The good news is that, by training your core muscles, you will be strengthening the muscles that hold up your back and automatically improving your posture.

RIGHT Good posture will make you stand more erect.

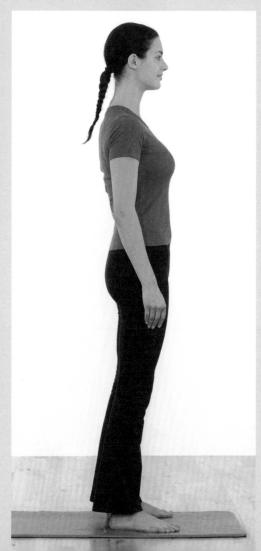

CORE MUSCLES

The muscles you need to know about for improving your core stability are those that are arranged around your torso.

ABDOMINAL MUSCLES

The abdominal muscles support the spine, protect internal organs, and enable you to sit, twist, and bend. The rectus abdominis is the muscle that runs from the bottom of your ribs to the pubic bone. It creates the "six-pack" look, but its actual purpose is to let you bend forward and sit up from a lying position. At the side of the torso are two diagonal muscles: the internal oblique and the external oblique. These bend the spine to the side and rotate it. Underneath the obliques lies the transversus abdominis, the deepest layer of muscles in your core. The transversus abdominis is responsible for trunk stability and pulls your stomach in tight.

BACK MUSCLES

There are two groups of back muscles that are important to core stability. The first group attaches between each of the vertebrae; the second along the whole length of the spine. The multifidus is the most important of these because it stiffens the spine.

PELVIC MUSCLES

These attach to the inside of the pelvis, forming a sling from the tailbone at the back to the pubic bone at the front. The pelvic muscles are vital for continence and help to maintain intra-abdominal pressure, which is key to stablization.

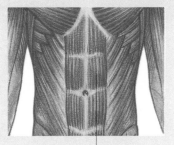

Rectus abdominis

TRUNK MUSCLES

The trunk muscles fall into two categories: inner (mainly responsible for stabilization) and outer (mainly responsible for movement). The inner unit muscles include the transversus abdominis, diaphragm, multifidus, and pelvic floor; the outer unit includes the obliques and spinal erectors. The inner and outer units work together to create spinal stability and enable subsequent movement.

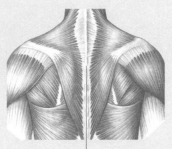

Multifidus

IMPROVING POSTURE

• Sleep on your back instead of on your front.

• Keep your head up and your shoulders back when walking.

• Bend your knees instead of your back when bending over to pick something up.

• Brace your abdominal muscles before lifting a heavy object; bend your knees instead of your back to pick it up and then carry it close to your body.

• If you tend to carry a lot in your shoulder bag or briefcase, you would be better off using a backpack to disperse the weight evenly.

Stand up straight and breathe

One of the great invisible advantages of improving your posture is that it will have a hugely beneficial effect on your breathing. This is a quick exercise that you can do at any time of day to pull yourself up straight and breathe better. It can help to do it in front of a mirror from time to time.

1 Stand tall with your feet pointing forward, about hips' width apart. Place your hands on your hips. Slowly bring your weight onto your heels, but leave the balls of your feet on the floor. Then bring your weight onto the balls of your feet, leaving your heels on the floor. Now raise your toes from the floor. Lower them back slowly.

3 Then push your hips forward, so that your buttocks come in and your pelvis tips backward.

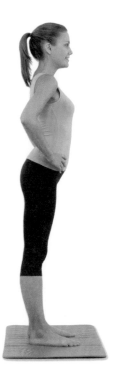

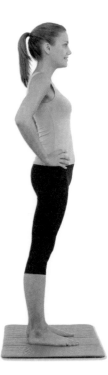

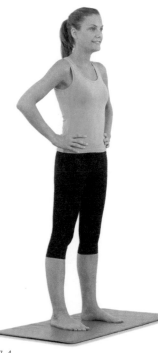

2 Place your hands on your hips. Stick your buttocks out so that your pelvis tips forward.

4 Find the midway point between these two positions: this is the neutral position for the pelvis. Pull up on your pelvic muscles and draw in the abdomen: this will help you to maintain the pelvis in neutral.

5 Bring your shoulders up toward your ears and hold them for a moment, then let them drop. Bring them forward, rounding the upper back and compressing the chest. Hold for a moment and then pull them backward, drawing the shoulder blades toward each other and down your back. Relax: Your shoulders should stay back and down.

6 Bring your head up, so that it is in line with the spine. It helps to imagine that there is a piece of string attached to the crown of your head; you can pull on a few hairs to feel the effect of this. Raise your chin upward and notice how the crown of your head tilts backward. Then drop the chin; the crown of your head drops forward. Bring the head into the midway neutral position so that the top of the head and the chin are parallel with the floor.

7 Go through the main points again: feet, pelvis, shoulders, and head, checking that each is in the right position.

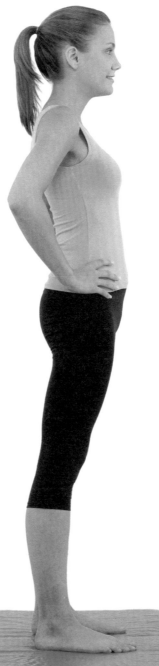

EXTRA TIP
Keep your knees "soft" instead of locked. To stand up straight, pull up on the thigh muscles instead of pushing the knees back.

Keep your body flexible

30

As we age, we become less supple, and joints, tendons, and muscles tend to stiffen up. It is particularly common for the thighs to tighten up, which can cause the hips and pelvis to rotate backward, resulting in bad posture. However, this problem can be effectively countered with these stretches.

1

SEATED HAMSTRING STRETCH

The hamstrings are the muscles running up the backs of the thighs to your buttocks. It is common for older people to have tight hamstrings, especially if they don't do enough exercise or, contrarily, if they do a lot of sport, which is why it's great to stretch them out. This stretch works both hamstrings at the same time, so you get double the benefit!

1 Sit down on the floor with your legs straight out in front of you, keeping your feet flexed. Sit up straight so that your back is not hunched and place your hands firmly on your hips.

3

2 Lean forward from the hips, letting your upper body drop down toward your feet. You can extend your arms and try to touch your toes, although if you do this, make sure that you don't curve your back.

3 Hold for ten seconds but don't bounce. Return to the starting position and repeat twice more.

76

INNER THIGH STRETCH

This stretch targets the muscles in the inner thighs, which are called the adductors. It's an easy way to stretch both the legs at once and is great if you combine it with a short meditation.

1 Sit on the floor with knees bent and soles of your feet pressed together so you're in a "frog" position. Hold the soles of your feet together with both hands.

2 Sit up, so your back is straight, and pull your stomach muscles in toward your spine.

3 Using the muscles in your inner thighs, push your knees down toward the floor. Make sure you don't bounce your knees.

4 When you've got your knees as far down as they can go, hold the stretch for ten seconds. Slowly release, then hold for two more sets of ten seconds.

EXTRA TIP
Make sure you don't curl your back. It makes it easier to reach the floor, but you'll be making the stretch far less effective.

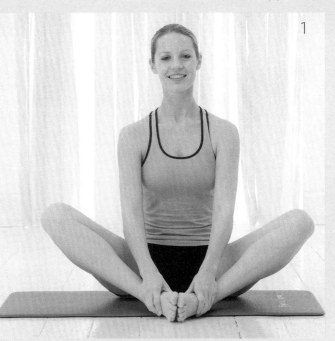

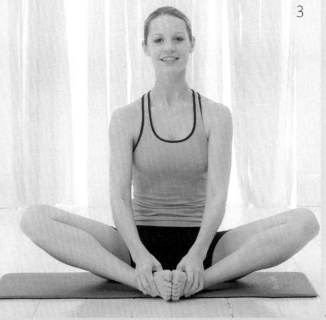

Stretch your backside

Your buttocks will lose muscle tone and tautness as the years pass, but that doesn't mean you have to put up with a sagging backside! There are a lot of great daily exercises you can do to keep your posterior perky and in the best possible shape. Here are two of the best.

PIRIFORMIS STRETCH

The piriformis muscles lie deep in the gluteal muscles (the ones in your buttocks). This is a good stretch to rejuvenate your buttocks after a long night's sleep. It will also help to keep it looking young and pert, but you do need to perform the exercise regularly in order to reap the maximum reward.

1 Lie on the floor on your back with both your knees bent, your feet flat on the floor, and palms down by your sides.

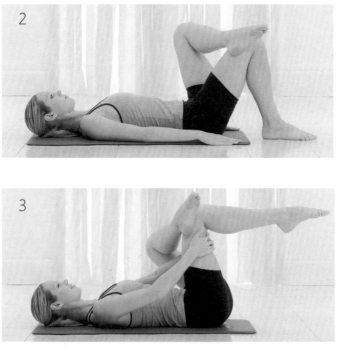

2 Lift your left leg off the ground and, rotating your leg from the hip, cross it over so the ankle of your left foot rests just above your right knee. Your left knee should be pointing to the left.

3 Grasp your right thigh with both hands and gently pull your right leg off the floor toward your chest. You will feel the stretch in the outside of your left leg.

4 Hold for two sets of seven seconds on your left leg and then repeat with the right leg.

BEND AND STRETCH

This is a tried and tested stretch that targets all the muscles at the back of the thighs and in the buttocks. Look forward toward the toes of your extended leg while you are doing the stretch, because it will inspire you to go as far as you can.

1 Stand a large step away from the front of a chair, with feet hips' width apart.

2 Lift your right leg and rest your right foot firmly on the seat of the chair. Your hands should be on your hips.

3 Bend over from the waist, and reach out to touch the toes of your right foot with both hands. You should feel the stretch in your right buttock and thigh.

4 Hold for two sets of seven seconds on your right leg, without bouncing, and then repeat with the left leg.

3

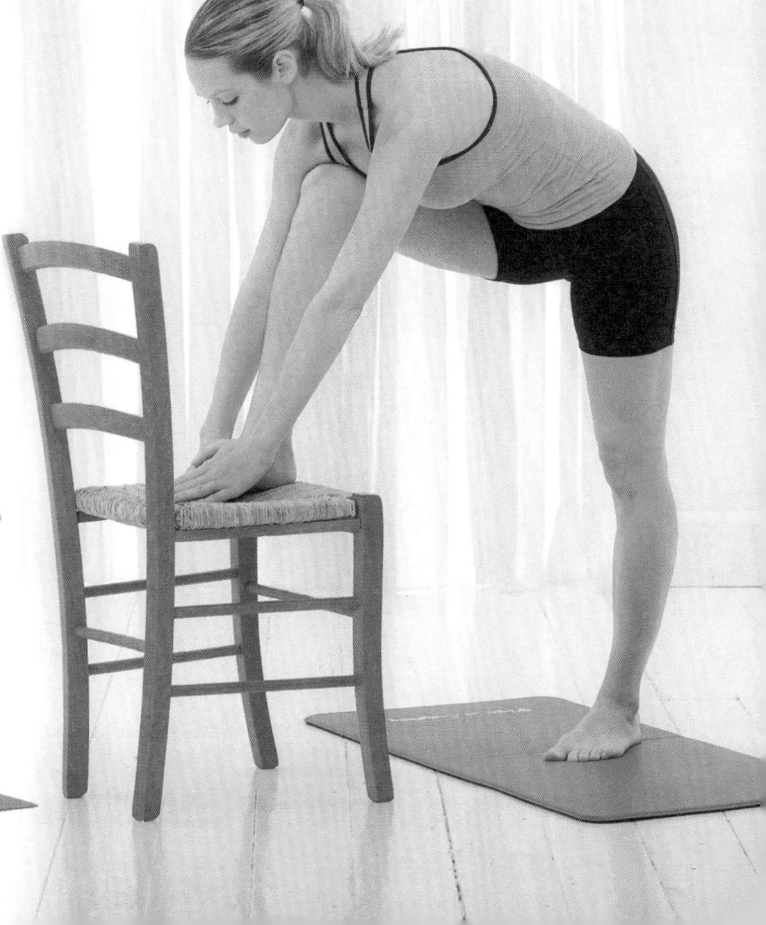

2

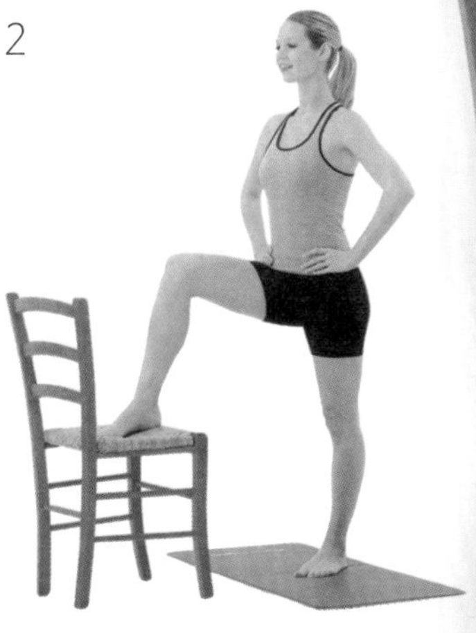

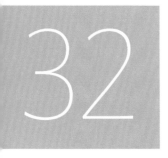

Work your calves & ankles

Calves and ankles can become tight and inflexible through both underuse and overuse. However, like all muscles, they lose some of their tone and suppleness as part of the aging process. The best way to counter this, and to keep your legs looking and feeling young, is to work them hard with stretches.

1

2

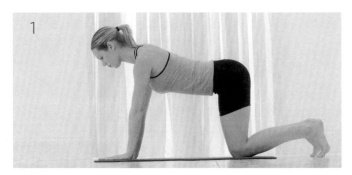

CALF STRETCH

If you do a lot of running or walking, you may find that your calves feel tight and inflexible. Contrarily, they might feel like this due to lack of exercise! This stretch will help them feel loose and tension-free.

1 Get down on the floor on your hands and knees, with your knees resting directly below your hips and your hands below your shoulders. Curl your toes under so they are resting on the floor.

2 Push up off the floor with both hands and straighten your legs, pushing your buttocks into the air. Your elbows and knees should be soft.

3 Try to lower your heels gently to the floor. Hold for three sets of ten seconds, returning to the start position in between.

PUSH-OFF CALF STRETCH

You usually see joggers doing this stretch before a big run—that's because it's a really good way of performing a controlled calf stretch that targets the gastrocnemius muscle (the big muscle at the back of the calf). To get the best stretch possible, make sure your full weight is shifted toward the wall.

1 Stand at arm's length from the wall, with your feet shoulder-width apart.

2 Extend your right leg out in front of you and bend your right knee.

3 Place the palms of your hands, at shoulder height, flat against the wall.

4 Take one step back with your left leg and, keeping it straight, press your heel firmly into the floor. You should feel the stretch in the calf of your left leg. Keep your hips facing the wall and your rear leg and spine in a straight line.

5 Hold the stretch for two sets of seven seconds, then repeat with the other leg.

4

2

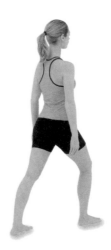

81

33 Keep your stomach lean

Your stomach and waist are two areas that might well require greater attention to keep them looking young, trim, and lean. Try these two basic stretches. Pull your stomach muscles in while you exercise—it will stop your back from arching. Also, as with all stretches, don't bounce during the exercises.

OBLIQUE STRETCH

This is an easy way to give the muscles in your waist a really good stretch. As you walk your hands around to get into position, you may not be able to reach your knees but that's fine—just go as far around as you can comfortably.

1 Get down on the floor on all fours with your knees resting directly below your hips and your hands below your shoulders.

2 Keeping your knees where they are, walk both your hands around to your right-hand side to meet your knees, so you are twisting from the waist. You should feel the stretch down your left-hand side. Hold the stretch for ten seconds, then walk the hands back around to the starting position. Repeat the movement so that you also stretch around to the left.

TWIST

The Twist is another great way of stretching out your obliques. This smooth movement will help you develop long and lean muscles to support a trim waist. You're only supposed to feel a subtle stretch, so don't make the mistake of twisting around too far in order to feel a greater one.

1 Stand with feet hips' width apart. Your feet should be flat on the floor and toes should be facing forward.

2 Extend both arms out to the sides at shoulder height.

3 Keeping your arms straight, gently rotate from the hip around to the left. Your hips and pelvis should remain facing forward.

4 Hold the position for two sets of seven seconds, until you feel the stretch in your waist. Slowly return to the starting position and then repeat on your right side.

3

Stretch your arms & chest

A key part of staying and looking young is keeping the skin and muscles of your arms and chest toned and supple. The two exercises featured on these pages will help you to relax and keep your upper body feeling strong and healthy as well as looking good. It is important to do the stretches regularly.

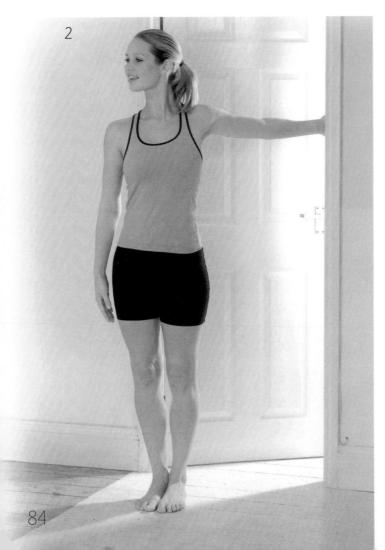

2

INNER ARM STRETCH

This targets all the muscles in your upper arms—you'll be surprised at how easy it is to feel the stretch.

1 Stand in an open doorway, with your abs tight and body straight.

2 Hold onto the doorjamb with your left hand just below shoulder level, or as high as is comfortable. Take a big step forward so your left arm is extended out behind you. Keeping your hips facing forward and your head and neck in line with your spine, rotate your upper body to the right until you feel the stretch in your left arm. Lean forward to feel a greater stretch.

3 Hold for two sets of seven seconds then turn around, step forward, and repeat the stretch with your right arm.

SEASHELL STRETCH

This stretch is great at targeting the muscles in your shoulders as well as your back. Just sit back and relax and you will feel the beneficial effects of the stretch.

1 Get down on the floor on your hands and knees. Sit back onto your calves, so your backside is resting on your heels. Make sure your neck and head are relaxed and that you are looking down toward the floor.

2 Stretch your arms out in front of you so that your hands and fingertips are spread on the floor.

3 Walk your hands as far forward as you can until you can feel the stretch in the middle of your back.

4 Hold the stretch for three sets of ten seconds.

1

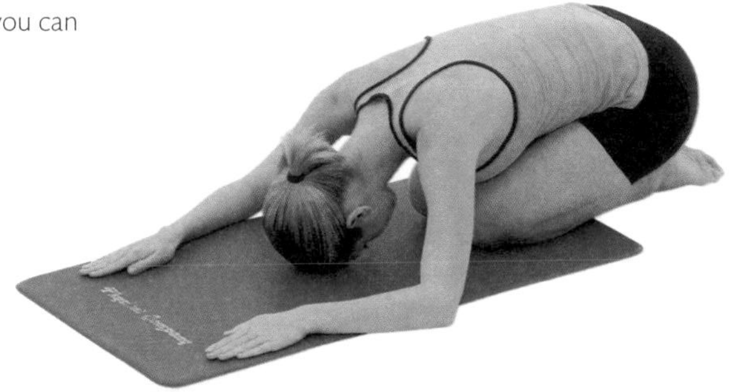

3

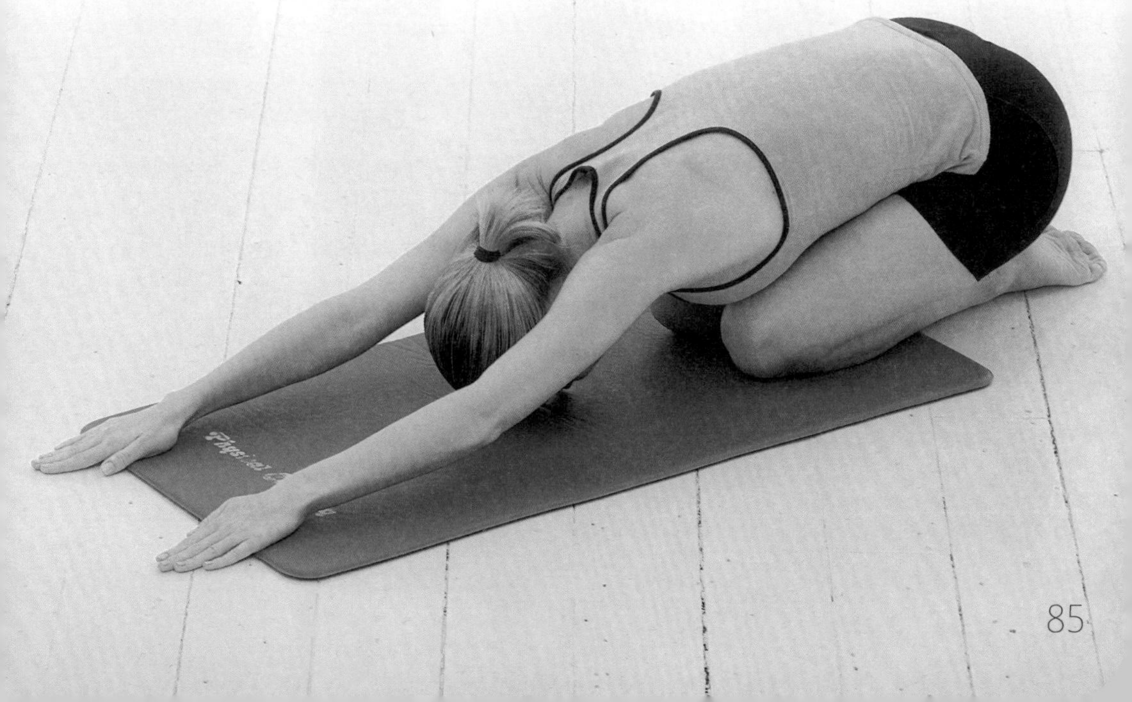

35

Relax your back & neck

It is important to stretch out the back and neck regularly to reduce tension and diminish stiffness. The muscles in your back and neck are the most likely to feel the effects of stress, so keeping them in good shape will make you feel better as well as automatically improving your posture.

WAIST AND LOWER SPINE

This is a great way of targeting your lower back muscles and really stretching them out thoroughly. If you do it slowly and gently, it can even be good at soothing lower back problems.

1 Lie on the floor on your back with your legs straight out and your right arm extended out to the side.

2 Bending your right leg, grip your knee with your left hand, and bring it over to your left-hand side so it gets as close to the floor as is comfortable.

3 Hold the stretch for two sets of seven seconds with a brief pause between. Repeat on your right side.

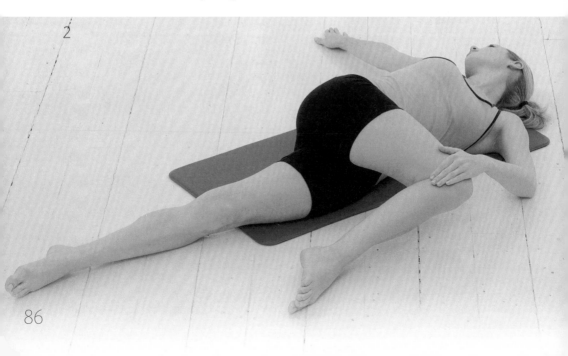

2

NECK STRETCHES

This is a great substitute for a neck massage. It really helps to get your muscles loose, warm, and stretched. Plus, it's much safer than rolling your neck, because it puts less of a strain on the surrounding muscles.

1 Stand up straight with feet hips' width apart. Relax your shoulders and look straight ahead of you.

2 Start the stretch by slowly lowering your chin to your chest. Hold for a few seconds while you feel the stretch across the back of your neck and then gently raise your head so it's back in the starting position.

3 Next, rotate your head to the right and hold for a few seconds, then rotate your head to the left. Hold for a few seconds, then return to the start position so you are looking straight ahead.

4 Repeat the sequence three times, until the 30 seconds are up.

2

3

3

Tone your legs

36

We can't all be blessed with slim, firm, and sexy legs, but toning them up and keeping them in the best possible condition will definitely make you feel good. Of course, no matter how they look, your legs have to carry you around, so if you want to feel young and vital, you need young and vital legs!

2

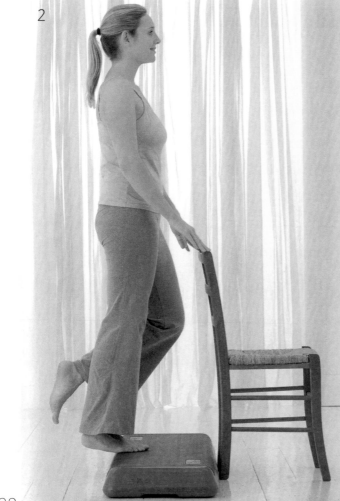

STANDING CALF RAISES

The calf muscles are hard to target, although studies have shown that walking in high heels can help to tone them up! To get really sexy, shapely calves, we recommend you try this exercise instead.

1 Stand with both feet near the edge of a raised object, such as a stair or a big chunky book. Place the ball of your right foot on the edge of the raised object, letting your heel extend off the edge.

2 Hold onto a wall or a chair for support and, lifting your left leg into the air slightly by bending at the knee, gently let your right heel drop down until you feel the stretch in your calf. Keep your back straight, your head up, and your right leg straight.

3 Rise up onto your right toe as high as you can and hold for a second while flexing the calf muscle.

4 Carefully return to the starting position, then repeat with the left leg.

SUPERMAN

You need to have a good sense of balance to do this exercise, so if you don't get it right first time, be patient. It's great for increasing core stability and endurance in the joints, as well as working the core muscles in your thighs.

1

2

1 Get down on the floor on all fours.

2 Contract your abs. Extend your right arm out in front of you and your left leg out behind you, keeping them as straight as you can without locking your elbow or knee. Engage your abdominal muscles to help stop your back from arching—it will reduce any risk of injury. You will feel the muscles working in the thigh of your extended leg. To increase the effects, try pointing your toes—it will make you tense your muscles harder. Keep your head and neck in line with your back to make sure you're not twisting your neck.

3 Slowly return to the start position and repeat with the opposite leg and arm.

37

Firm up your backside

Perhaps surprisingly, human beings are often subconsciously influenced by the appearance of someone else's backside. Firm, well-toned, and muscular buttocks denote virility and send powerful subliminal messages about the sexuality of the owner. They also indicate youth, health, and vigor.

REAR LEG RAISE

This exercise will help to strengthen and tone both the gluteus maximus (the major muscles in the buttocks, which are also known as the glutes) and also the lower back.

1 Lie face down on the floor with your forehead resting on the backs of your hands. Make sure your spine is in line with your neck.

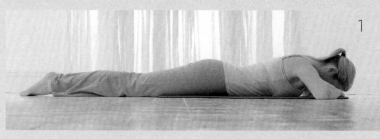

1

2 Squeeze your buttocks—it will make the exercise more effective. Then, engage your abdominal muscles and gently lift your right leg off the floor until you feel the muscles working in your buttocks. Keep your leg straight and your knee soft. You shouldn't feel any pain in your lower back.

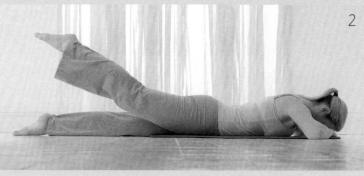

2

3 Lower your right leg back into the starting position, then repeat the movement with your left leg and again with your right, and so on until the 30 seconds are up.

LUNGE

In this exercise, shifting your core body weight to the front means that the muscles in your buttocks will bear most of the brunt. Lunging is great for strengthening as well as toning the muscles and is a firm favorite among personal fitness trainers. This exercise will really keep your buttocks looking and feeling young!

1 Stand with your feet hips' width apart. Rest your hands on your hips or by your sides.

2 Step forward with your right leg, bending your knee so that your thigh is almost at a right angle to the floor. Your right foot should be flat on the floor. Your left leg should be slightly bent at the knee and the ball of your left foot should be resting on the floor behind you, with your heel slightly in the air.

3 Hold for a second, then push off the floor with your right foot and return to the starting position.

4 Repeat the movement with alternate legs until the 30 seconds are up.

2

38

Work your stomach muscles

Do you worry about the state of your belly? We bet you do. Do you think it sticks out too much, or looks saggy or wobbly? A well-toned stomach is a youthful stomach, that will look good both in clothes or exposed on the beach or in the bedroom. Follow these exercises for supertight abdominals!

THE PUSH-UP

This doesn't sound or look too taxing, but, if you do it right, you'll find that it's one of the most intense exercises in this book and very effective for toning the abdominal muscles.

1 Lie on the floor on your front, resting your forehead on the backs of your hands.

2 Keeping your elbows bent, slide your hands across the floor, rotating from the shoulders, until you find your perfect "push-up" position at either side of your chest.

3 Curl your toes underneath you and push up off the floor with your hands. Keep your elbows soft to stop them from locking, and keep your neck and head relaxed and in line with your spine.

4 Hold the pose for ten seconds, then gently lower yourself back down to the floor again. Remember to breathe during the exercise.

2

3

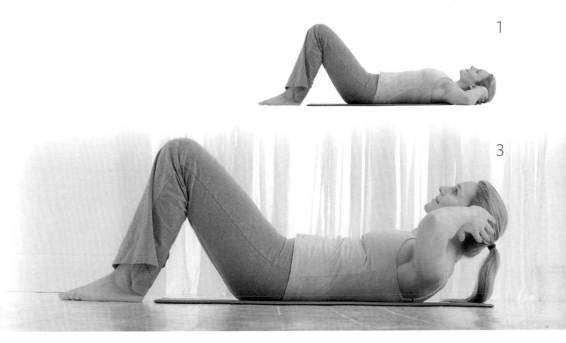

1

3

CRUNCHES

This is an intense workout for your stomach muscles and a great way of getting a washboard-flat stomach.

1 Lie on the floor, with your knees bent and feet (apart) flat on the floor in line with your hips. Make sure your lower back is pressed into the floor. Put your hands behind your head to support your neck.

2 Engage your stomach muscles, by pulling your abs toward your spine, and lift your upper body off the floor as far as you can without arching your lower back. You may find that you can't get up very high, but it's the effort of moving that counts, so make sure that you're pushing yourself as hard as you comfortably can. With practice, you may be able to sit up completely.

3 When you can't go any further, pause for one second. Then gently lower yourself back down into the starting position and repeat.

39

Tone your chest & back

Here are a couple of handy toning exercises that are great for your entire torso—both front and back. If you do these stretches regularly, they will keep you looking and feeling strong and upright, while working wonders for your bosom without the need for enhancements or push-up bras!

WALL PUSH-UP

This is like a standing push-up and is great for toning the muscles in the chest, especially the pectoral muscles (known as the pecs), which can be found underneath your bust.

1 Stand around 2 feet (60 cm) away from the wall, feet hips' width apart and legs straight. Make sure your knees are soft.

2 Lean forward and place your palms flat against the wall.

3 Bend your arms at the elbows and bring your chest toward the wall.

4 Squeeze the muscles in your chest and push off from the wall so you are standing back in the start position.

3

MOY COMPLEX

This exercise is also known as the "row, rotate, and press" and is a great way to tone the muscles in your back, without having to use the complicated machinery that you find in the gym.

1 Sit on the edge of a chair with a dumbbell or a can of soup in each hand.

2 Bend over from the waist so that your chest is resting on your knees. Make sure your head and neck are relaxed, so that you're looking down toward the floor.

3 Start with your hands resting on the floor, with elbows slightly bent, then bend your arms and bring your hands up to shoulder level.

4 Rotate your wrists and extend your arms out in front of you so that they're parallel to the floor.

5 Retrace your steps so you're back in the Step 2 position, then repeat the movement.

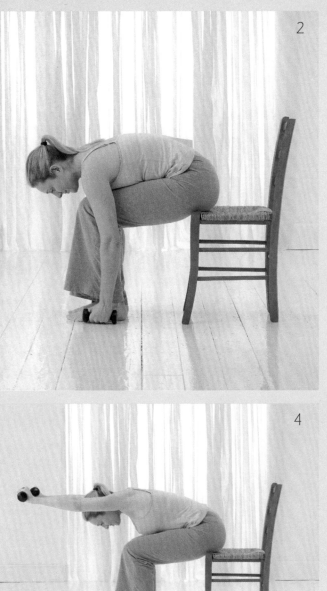

95

40

Exercise your triceps

There are numerous benefits to keeping your arms in good shape. If you exercise them regularly, not only will they look good, they will be powerful and efficient as well. For centuries, arm strength has been associated with youth and vitality in both sexes, so why not keep yours fit and strong?

TRICEPS SQUEEZE BACK

This is an easy-to-perform standing exercise that will tone through the back of your upper arms, creating a long, toned triceps muscle and banishing any wobbly arms. The other great thing with this exercise is that it also stretches your chest muscles, which helps promote good posture.

1 Stand with good posture and your knees slightly bent. Hold the weights keeping your arms by your side, with your palms facing away from you backward.

2 Lift your chest and pull your shoulders back.

3 Lift both arms directly behind you, and feel this working through your triceps. Hold your arms at the highest point, then slowly lower back to the start position.

1

3

TRICEPS PONY TAIL

This standing triceps exercise is one of the best ways to tone flabby upper arms.

1 Stand with good posture. Bend your knees slightly and pull in your stomach. Place a weight in your right hand, then extend the right arm straight up and support it with the other arm. Keep a good posture and your abdominal muscles pulled in.

2 Now simply bend at the elbow of your extended arm so that the weight comes up by your upper back. Slowly straighten the arm back up to the start position. Do all your repetitions on one arm and then repeat on the other arm.

1

2

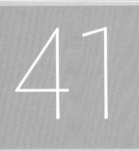

Tighten your biceps

These seated exercises will work wonders to improve your muscle tone and general posture. Like all the exercises in this chapter, they need to be performed regularly in order to be effective, but they really do work. Banish arm wobble and flabby biceps with these simple seated workouts.

BENT-OVER ARM SHAPER
This seated exercise will target your arms and your upper back muscles and improve your upper body flexibility

1 Using a weight in each hand, sit on the edge of your chair, bent over, with arms hanging down, feet slightly apart.

2 Keep your abdominal muscles pulled in to stop you from collapsing your back onto your legs.

3 Lift your arms out to the sides, up to shoulder level, squeezing your shoulder blades together. Lower the arms and repeat.

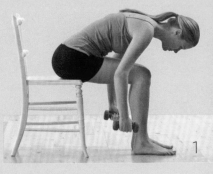

1

3

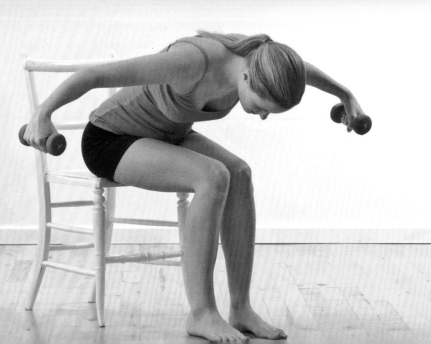

BICEPS CURL

This exercise focuses on working the biceps muscle through a full range of motion.

1 Sit leaning forward with your legs slightly spread and your left hand on your left thigh.

2 Hold a weight in your right hand and at arm's length, your elbow resting against the inside of your knee.

3 From this position, slowly lift your arm upward to make an L shape.

4 With the weight at knee height, slowly lift your arm up toward your chest. Hold for a second, lower, then slowly go all the way back to the start position. Repeat on the other arm.

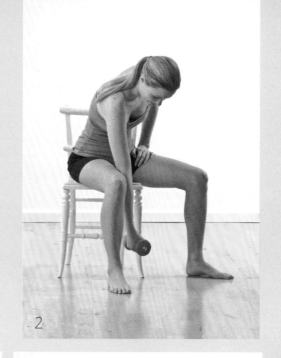

2

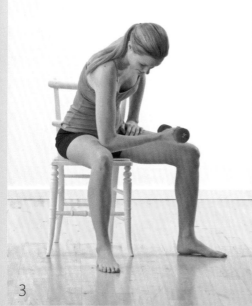

3

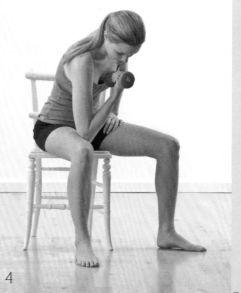

4

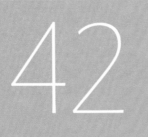

Exercise your arms

You wouldn't have thought that getting arm fit would involve doing exercises on the floor, but these somewhat more challenging routines will have your arms feeling better than they have done for ages in no time. You should try the other exercises and work on your general fitness before doing these.

FLOOR ARM LIFT

This is a challenging exercise but it is fantastic for sculpting your upper arms as it really works your triceps.

1 Sit on the mat with your legs straight and together. Place your hands, fingertips forward, just behind your hips, and point your toes.

2 Pull in your abdominal muscles, straighten your arms (hands should be under your shoulders), and lift your hips off the floor until your body is aligned from shoulders to toes. Keep looking forward.

3 Hold the position for a second, then slowly lower.

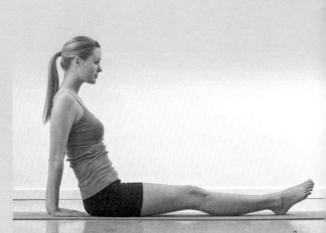

1

2

SUPERWOMAN ARMS

This will tone through your shoulders and biceps, while working to improve your shoulder joint flexibility.

1 Kneel on the mat on all fours, with your wrists directly under your shoulders and your knees under your hips on the mat. Keep your abdominal muscles contracted. Holding a small weight, lift up one arm so that it is in line with your shoulder.

2 Now slowly bend the arm back so that your elbow is then in line with your shoulder. Hold, then gently release back to a straight arm and repeat. Do all your repetitions on one arm and then repeat on the other arm.

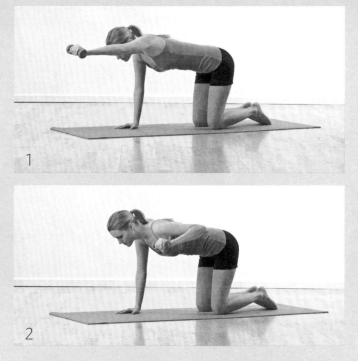

1

2

BACK EXTENSIONS

It is important for great upper body posture to have strong back muscles. This will help keep you strong and upright while also toning through your upper arms.

1 Lie face down on the mat and place your fingertips by the side of your head.

2 Contract your abdominal muscles and keep them contracted throughout the exercise.

3 Squeeze the back to lift the chest a little way off the floor. Hold for a second. Then slowly lower back down.

3

43

Firm up your stomach

A flat and firm stomach is a surefire aid to a youthful appearance. Whether clothed or naked, it will make you feel better and more confident about your body. It is not as hard as you might think to get one, either. Practice the following exercises regularly and reap the rewards in no time.

SEATED KNEE LIFT

This seated exercise will work your rectus abdominis—the muscle that runs down the front of your stomach. Make sure your movements are controlled and flowing.

1 Sit on the edge of a chair with your knees bent and pressed together and your feet flat on the floor. Hold onto the sides of the chair, then tighten your stomach muscles.

2 Lean back slightly and lift your feet a few inches off the ground, keeping your knees bent and pressed together.

3 Slowly pull your knees in toward your chest and curl your upper body forward. Then lower your feet to the floor. Rest for a count of three before you do any repetitions.

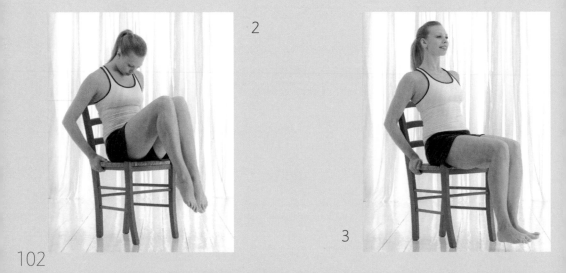

2

3

SPINE ROTATION

This exercise gently mobilizes your spine, preparing it for harder exercises to come.

1 Sit forward on a chair with your back straight and your hands resting on your thighs. Your knees should be over your ankles.

2 Tighten your abdominal muscles. Keeping your hips and knees forward, slowly rotate your upper body to the left until you can put both hands on the back of the chair. Hold for a count of ten, then return to the center. Repeat the exercise, twisting to the right.

DON'T EXERCISE IF...

- You are feeling unwell—your body will need all its strength to fight off any infection.
- You have an injury—you might make things worse.
- You have an ongoing medical condition or are on medication—consult your doctor before embarking on any course of exercise.
- You've just had a big meal.
- You've been drinking alcohol.

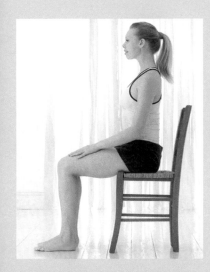

1

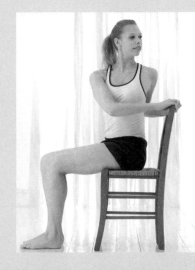

2

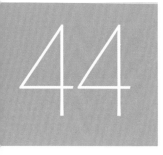

Get a taut, flat stomach

The following exercises need a slightly higher level of fitness to be performed properly and require deep, controlled breathing throughout. They will improve the firmness and strength of your abdominal muscles while hopefully giving you a sense of calm and inner peace due to the deep breathing required.

BELLY TIGHTENER

This is also known as abdominal hollowing and helps to shorten the abdominal muscles, which is good for your posture and creates the appearance of a flatter stomach. Exercising in this position means you are working against gravity, making your muscles work even harder. Remember to keep your elbows soft, not locked.

1 Kneel down on all fours (the "box" position) with your hands shoulders' width apart, your elbows slightly bent, and your knees under your hips. Keep your head in line with the rest of your body and look down at the floor, making sure that your chin isn't tucked into your chest.

2 Relax your abdominal muscles, then slowly draw in your navel toward your spine.

3 Hold the muscles in for a count of ten, then slowly relax. Breathe slowly and steadily throughout this exercise.

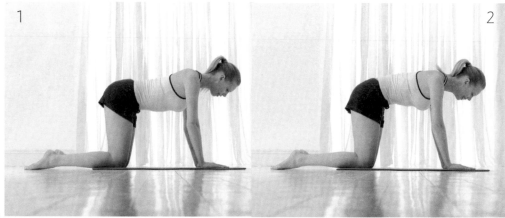

EASY PUSH-UP (TENSION HOLD)

Holding your body in a three-quarters plank shape strengthens the deep transverse muscles that cross the stomach area. Keeping your knees on the floor makes this exercise much easier than the traditional push-up, which you can progress to when you feel ready.

1 Adopt a traditional push-up position, but keep your knees on the floor and your feet in the air. Your fingers should point forward, your elbows should stay straight but not locked, your head should be in line with your body, and your feet should be together. Keep your shoulder blades drawn into your back and make sure you don't dip in the middle or raise your backside in the air.

2 Hold this position for a count of ten, breathing regularly throughout.

HOW TO BREATHE PROPERLY

Breathing is something we all take for granted, but most of us only use the top third of our lungs. Learn to breathe properly and it's probably the best thing you can do for your overall health, because oxygen nourishes and replenishes all your body's cells. Abdominal breathing is a technique that enables you to breathe more deeply. It uses the diaphragm, the sheet of muscle forming the top of the abdomen, to help the lungs inflate and deflate effortlessly. Breathe in slowly through your nose, and notice how the top of the abdomen rises as you do so. Hold the breath for a few seconds, then breathe out slowly through your mouth.

1

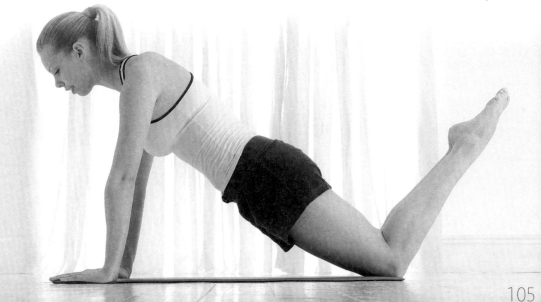

Strengthen your abdominals

These exercises will tighten the abdominal muscles without putting any strain on your back. They're a simple way to tone and strengthen your abdominal muscles. Always use a proper exercise mat designed for the purpose and clear plenty of space on the floor before you begin.

SIMPLE PELVIC TILT

This easy exercise is particularly good for firming excess belly flab.

1 Lie on your back with your knees bent and feet flat on the floor, hips' width apart, and your spine in neutral. Rest your arms by your sides, palms facing the floor, and tighten your abdominal muscles.

2 Press your lower back down into the floor and gently tilt your pelvis so that the pubic bone rises, then tilt it back down.

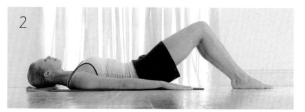

3 Repeat several times, using a slow, steady rhythm.

LEG SLIDE

Another easy exercise for tightening your stomach muscles.

1 Lie on your back with your knees bent, your feet flat on the floor, and your arms by your sides, palms facing the floor.

2 Tighten your abdominal muscles by gently pulling in your navel toward your backbone.

3 Gently tilt your pelvis so that the pelvic bone rises.

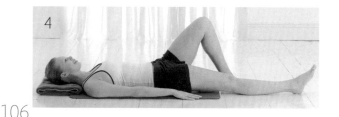

4 Raising the toes of one foot, breathe out while sliding your leg forward as far as it will go, with your heel on the floor.

LOWER ABDOMINAL RAISE

This is a harder exercise that will really work your deep abdominal muscles. If it seems easy, then you're not doing it properly!

1 Lie on your back with your knees bent, feet flat on the floor, and hips' width apart. Make sure your spine is in neutral. Keep your arms by your sides with the palms facing upward.

2 Lift your legs into the air at an angle of 90 degrees to your body.

3 Tighten your abdominal muscles and slowly lower one foot to the floor, then bring it back up again.

4 Repeat this exercise using the other leg.

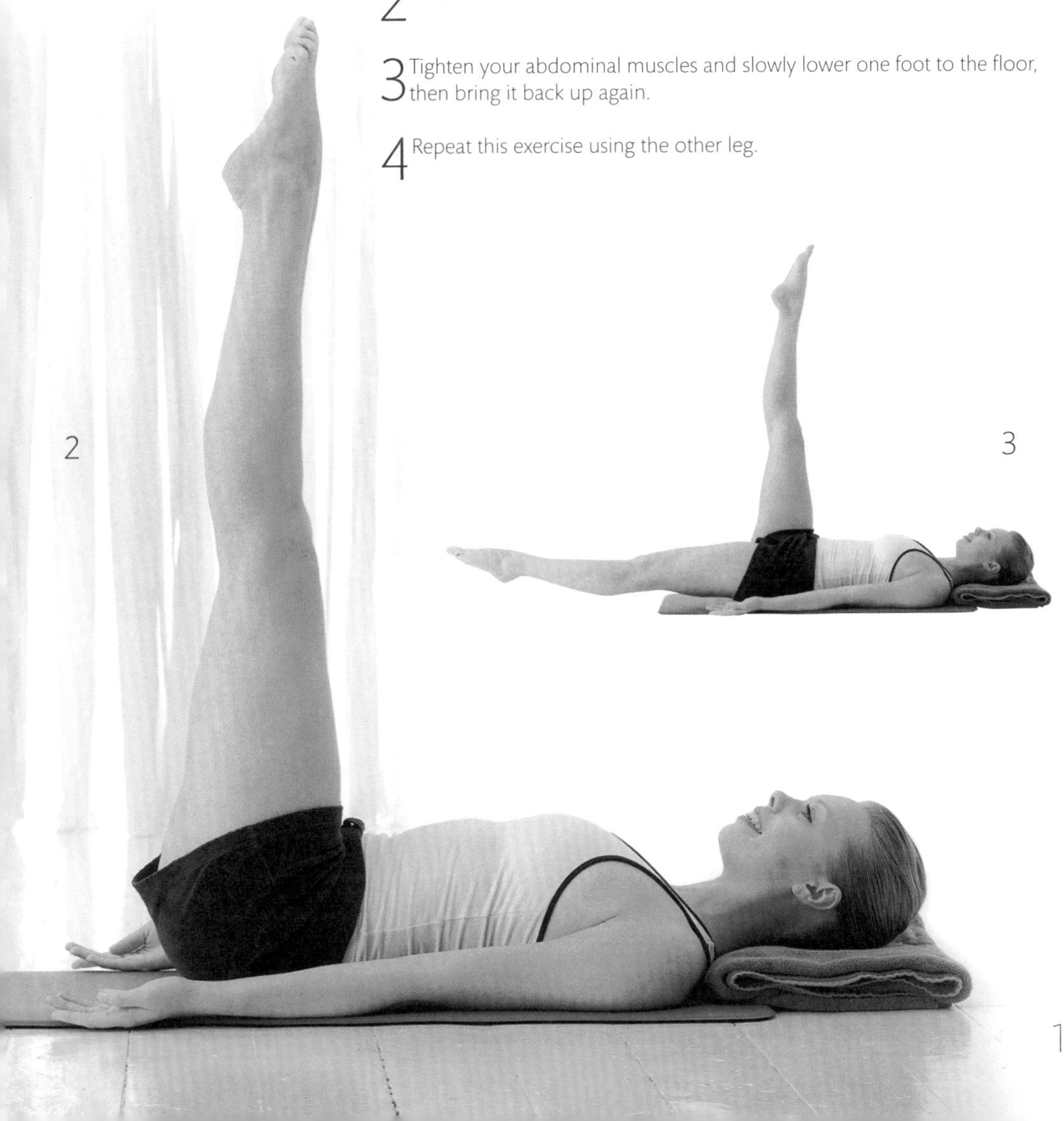

2

3

107

46

Exercise your thighs & hips

Even if you're office-bound for a large part of the day or spend a lot of time traveling, you can still sneak in a few exercises to keep your hips and thigh muscles toned. You'll need a straight-back, sturdy chair for these exercises—not one on wheels. Do these as often as possible to keep your legs feeling young.

SEATED LEG EXTENSION

This easy exercise is great for toning the quadriceps, the muscles at the front of your thighs. To make this harder, you can use ankle weights to strengthen the intensity of the exercise.

1 Sit up straight with good posture. Tighten your abdominal muscles by pulling in your navel toward your spine (which will protect your back muscles).

2 Press your knees together and straighten one leg. Hold and release. Do all your reps on one leg, then repeat the exercise on the other leg.

2

1

SIMPLE SEATED THIGH SQUEEZE

This tones and strengthens your inner thighs. Make this exercise harder by increasing the time of the squeeze and by using something with more resistance, such as a semi-inflated ball.

1 Sit up straight on a chair with your knees bent and feet together.

2 Place a cushion between your thighs.

3 Squeeze the cushion as hard as possible for a count of five, then release.

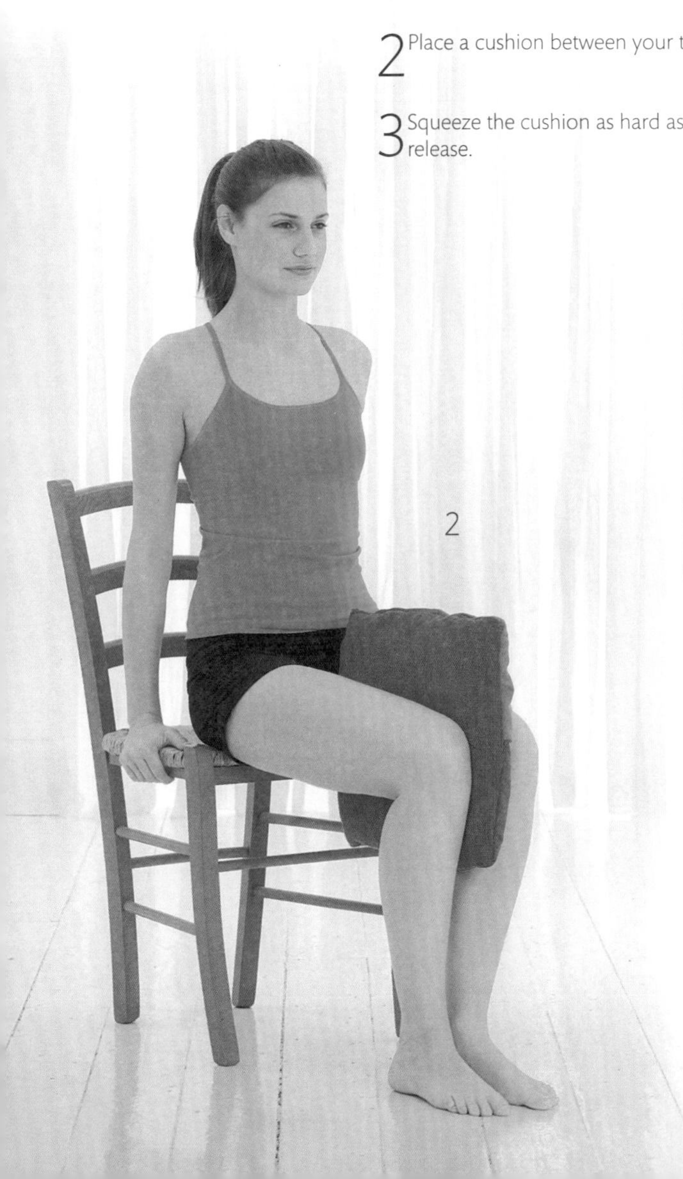

2

✳ TIP BOX

MAKING THE EFFORT
It's important to work at the right intensity if you're aiming to tone up your muscles—if you work out until it hurts, you may damage your muscles; put in too little effort and you won't notice any difference.

Strengthen your thighs & hips

Make sure that all exercises are performed slowly, carefully, and with your full attention. You need to concentrate on what you're doing and think about how your body is responding to any exercise. If an action hurts or you do it quickly, then you're not doing it properly.

BRIDGE WITH LEG LIFT

Lifting one leg strengthens the muscles at the back of the buttocks and thighs while increasing balance and control in your stabilizing muscles.

1 Lie on your back with your knees bent and feet slightly apart, and your arms at your sides.

2 Tighten your abdominal muscles by gently drawing in your navel toward your spine.

3 Curl your backside off the floor, lifting your pelvis until your knees, hips, and chest are in line.

4 Extend one leg, lift it level with the knee, then lower to the floor. Do all your reps on one leg, then repeat on the other leg.

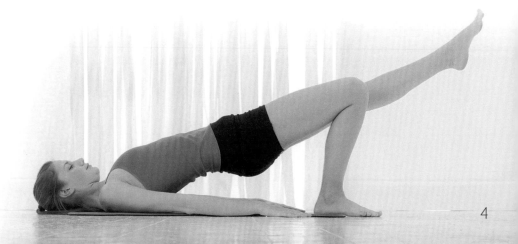

4

ONE-LEG BUTTOCK CLENCHER

This is a harder exercise that will really work your gluteals.

1 Lie on your back with your knees bent and your feet flat on the floor, slightly apart. Keep your arms by your sides, palms facing downward.

2 Place your left foot onto your right knee.

3 Tighten your abdominal muscles to support your back.

4 Press your lower back down into the floor and gently tilt your pelvis forward so that the pubic bone rises. Lift your hips off the floor and squeeze your buttock muscles, then release. Do all your reps on one leg, then repeat on the other leg.

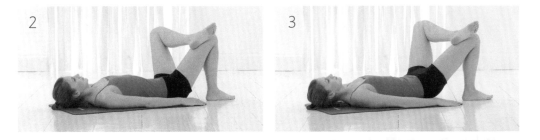

BUTTOCK WALKING

This exercise is wonderful for keeping your backside trim and strengthening the buttock muscles. The floor is a good option because a hard surface is more taxing, but beware of carpet burn or splinters from old wooden floors.

1 Sit up straight with your legs stretched out in front of you. Cross your arms so that your hands are resting on your shoulders.

2 Breathe in and lengthen your spine. Breathe out, and breathe normally as you "walk" forward on your buttocks—ten steps forward, ten steps back, to form one rep. Repeat as often as you can.

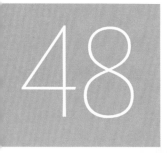

Improve your balance

As well as exercising your hip and thigh muscles, these leg lifts help to improve your balance. You will need to hold onto the back of a chair or a table for support for all these exercises. Keep all your movements smooth and fluid and move only as far as is comfortable for your body.

3

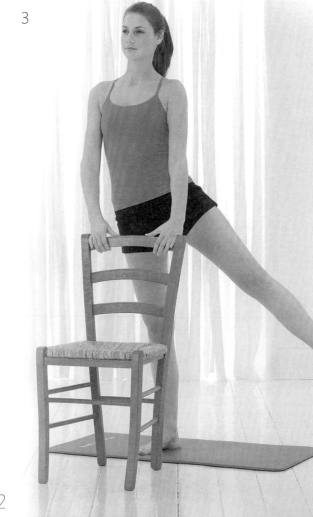

LATERAL LEG RAISE

This exercise helps to tone and tighten your outer thigh muscles and your hips, as well as improve your balance.

1 Stand up straight with good posture, hands by your sides, and feet together, holding onto the back of a chair with both hands for balance.

2 Tighten your abdominal muscles by gently drawing in your navel toward your spine (which will protect your lower back muscles).

3 Simply raise one leg out to the side about 45 degrees. Keep your toes pointing forward and hold for a count of three. Relax and do all your reps on one leg, then repeat using the other leg.

FRONT LEG RAISE

This exercise strengthens and tones the front of your thighs (quadriceps) and increases your hip flexibility. It also helps with your balance.

1 Stand up straight with your feet together and hold onto the back of a chair sideways with your left hand to balance. Tighten your stomach muscles.

2 With your left leg slightly bent, raise your right leg out in front of you as far as is comfortable.

3 Hold for a count of three.

4 Lower and do all your reps on one leg, then repeat on the other leg.

2

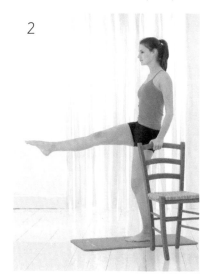

3

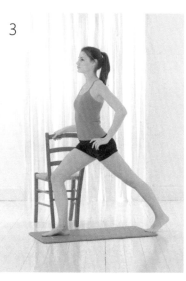

REAR LEG RAISE

This strengthens and tones the buttocks, lower back, back of hips, and hamstrings. It also helps with your balance. For best results, keep your buttocks tensed throughout—it's harder but better for you in the long run!

1 Stand up straight with your feet together and use your right hand to hold onto the back of a chair sideways to help you balance.

2 Pull in your stomach muscles to support your back and tighten your buttock muscles.

3 Take your left leg back, and touch the floor with your toes. Hold this position for a count of three, then return to the start. Do all your reps on one leg, then repeat on the other leg.

113

49

Strengthen your back

A strong back is the key to a healthy, lithe young body. The stretches in the next few pages are suitable for most people. However, they are general exercises, so it is important that you take individual advice on whether they are suitable for you if you have had any back pain or back problems in the past.

STRETCH UP

Doing a few gentle movements in the morning will stretch out the spine and help to get your circulation going, sending blood and oxygen to your muscles and ligaments.

1 Take a few moments to stand and breathe deeply. Stand tall, with your feet hips' width apart, your arms by your sides.

2 Very slowly, bring your arms up in a wide circle and above your head. Don't exaggerate the movement; let it be natural.

3 Stretch one arm up, letting the elbow of the other arm bend slightly. Then stretch the other arm up in the same way. Repeat these alternate movements three or four times, as if you are pulling on a rope. Keep your head level throughout the exercise, looking straight ahead of you. To end, slowly circle the arms down again.

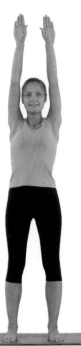

2

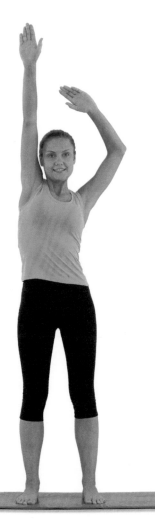

3

SHOULDER SHRUGS

Doing these easy shoulder shrugs regularly will reduce tension and improve your muscle tone.

1 Check that your head is held erect and level; pull your chin back and feel your neck lengthen. Then slowly bring your shoulders up toward your ears.

2 Let your shoulders slowly drop back down again. Keep your back relaxed as you do this three or four times.

3 Now rotate the shoulders in a clockwise direction three or four times. Then rotate them in the opposite direction three or four times.

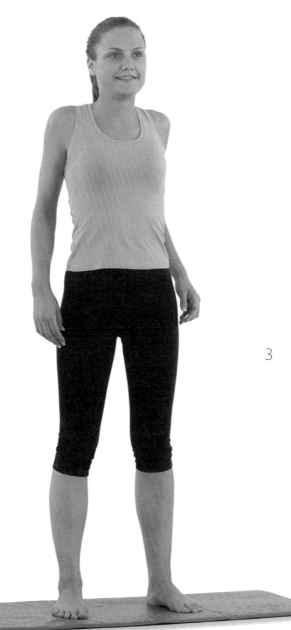

1

3

115

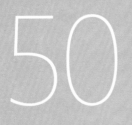

Improve your stance

Strengthening your back will help other areas of your body to become stronger, too. By following these exercises, the resulting improvements in your stance and posture will mean that your limbs and other parts of your physique will automatically fall into a better and healthier alignment.

SEATED TWIST

Like the supine twist, this exercise helps to improve the back's mobility in turning from side to side. It also feels really good.

1 Sit upright with your legs out in front of you. Bend your left leg, lift the foot, and place it on the mat so that it rests against the outside of your right calf. Rest your left elbow on your left knee and your left hand on your thigh.

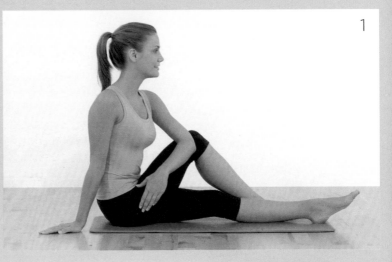

1

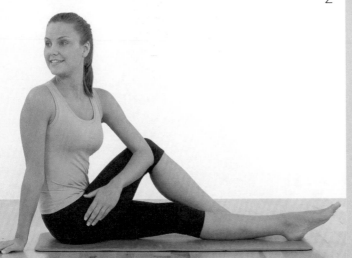

2

2 Breathe in and extend the spine upward. Breathe out and very slowly turn to the right. Hold for a count of five, breathing normally.

3 Breathing out, return to the central position. Then change the position of your legs and arms, and repeat on the other side. Repeat on both sides once more.

BACK ARCH

This useful and popular exercise helps to stretch the spine backward, countering the effects of slouching. Go only as far as feels comfortable. Stop immediately if you feel any pain.

1 Lie down on your front. Keep your legs together, tuck your toes under, and place your hands just under your shoulders (as if you were preparing to do a push-up).

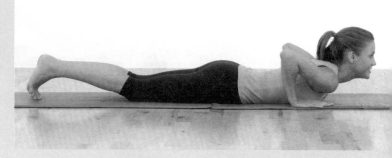

1

2 Very slowly straighten your arms, lifting your head and shoulders upward. Breathe in as you do so. Hold the position for a count of five, breathing, then slowly lower yourself back down.

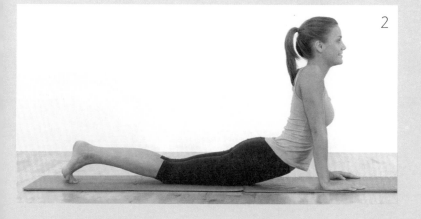

2

3 Repeat up to ten times. As you repeat the exercise, you may find that you can go a little farther each time. However, do not try to force your back up.

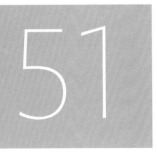

Keep your back supple

As the years pass, our muscles atrophy and become less supple. Those of the back are no exception. They need looking after and toning regularly to keep them young and working at full capacity. These final exercises in this chapter show you how to keep your back muscles strong and flexible.

SINGLE LEG LIFT

This exercise and the shoulder raise and double leg lift opposite help to strengthen the muscles of the back.

1 Lie on your front, legs together and arms folded so that you can rest your chin on them.

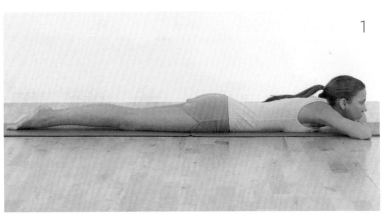

1

2

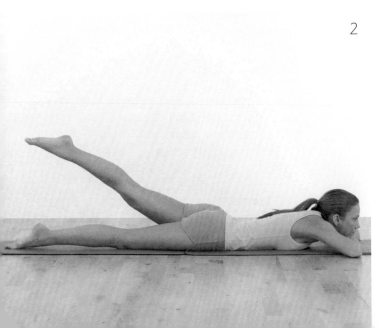

2 Very slowly, raise one leg as you breathe in. Keep it stretching back as you do so, with the toes pointing backward, but do not lock your knee. Lift the leg as far as you can without feeling strain in the back, then hold for a count of five, breathing normally. Bring the leg back down to the floor as you breathe out, and repeat up to ten times.

3 Do the same with the other leg, again lifting it only as far as feels comfortable. It doesn't matter if one leg lifts up higher than the other as long as it is comfortable.

SHOULDER RAISE AND DOUBLE LEG LIFT

The shoulder raise and double leg lifts are more difficult than the previous exercise, so you should only try them if you can do single leg lifts easily.

1 Lie on your front, legs together as in the single leg lifts and rest your head on a towel. This time bring your hands behind your back, placing the back of your left hand in the palm of your right, and rest them on your buttocks.

2 Breathe in and bring your shoulders off the ground. Keep looking at the floor, so that your head and neck stay in line with the spine. Hold for a count of five, then breathe out, as you lower yourself down to the floor again. Repeat up to ten times.

3 Remove the folded towel. Now place your arms by your sides, palms facing upward. Turn your head to one side so that you rest your face on the mat. Then breathe in and raise both legs off the floor simultaneously. Hold for a count of five, then breathe out and return to the floor. Repeat up to ten times.

1

2

3

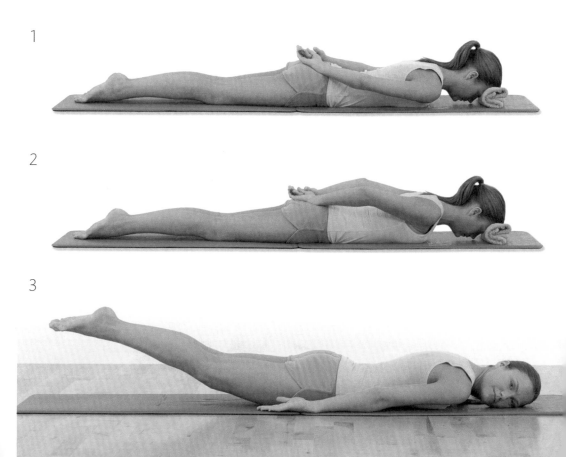

Focus on the face

Our faces say more about us to the outside world than probably anything else. If you want to project a young and fit image, then a well cared for, healthy, and happy face is a good place to start. You cannot change the face you were born with, but you can look after it and make the most of it. This chapter shows you how, with a blend of facial exercises, massages and cleansing and rejuvenating routines that will leave you looking and feeling fresh and youthful.

Introduction

How do you feel about your face? Are you happy with it? Does it reflect who you really are? Whatever the answers to these questions, chances are you want to make the best of it and keep it looking as young as possible. Follow the advice in this chapter and make the most of your unique face.

BEAUTIFUL SKIN

Beautiful skin is essential for making the most of your looks. Without it, all that carefully applied makeup will either turn patchy and blotchy, slide into lines and wrinkles, or disappear off your face in a shiny, oily mess. The simple truth is that most of us don't have beautiful skin. In fact, we don't even have so-called "normal" skin, with its plump, shiny texture, radiant glow, and minimal breakouts. Instead we have dry patches, oily patches, or irritated patches, and that means our skin doesn't always look or feel as good as it should. And the problems tend to get worse as you become older. However, the good news is that you don't have to put up with this. By knowing what kind of skin you have and how to treat it, you can solve your particular problems. Balance the levels of water and oil in your skin and you will create the state of harmony that is beautiful, perfect, "normal" skin. Read on and we will show you how—whatever your skin type.

THE BENEFITS OF GOOD FACIAL CARE

In this chapter, we start by showing you how to "wake up" and stimulate your face with a series of easy-to-follow exercises for all the facial muscles. We then offer you a complete set of facial treatments that show you how to love and pamper any kind of facial skin. Finally, we offer several facial massage and rejuvenation routines, guaranteed to bring a youthful glow back to your face, followed by helpful advice about the beneficial effects of light and sleep on your skin. Remember these basic antiaging tips in addition, and you should soon have a more youthful looking face:

- Moisturize thoroughly—a young looking, healthy face is a moist face. Find the best moisturizer for your face, apply it regularly, and stick with it.
- Don't stop at the jawbone—if you want to keep yourself looking young, remember to extend your treatments to your neck as well as your face.
- Plump up your pucker—dry, scaly lips are old-looking lips. Keep yours looking their best with regular applications of a good hydrating lip balm.
- Whiten your smile—it's easy to forget that your teeth are part of your face! Take years off your look by having your teeth whitened regularly.

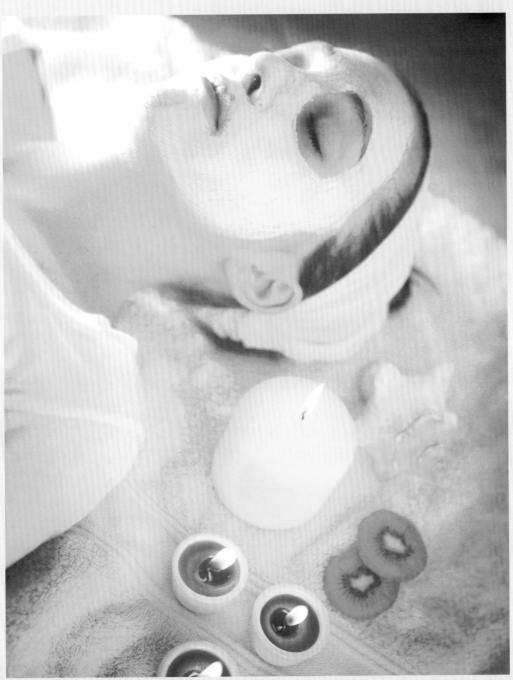

52

Wake up with facerobics

This antiaging routine is designed to improve skin texture and to rejuvenate slack tissue and sagging muscles. The first time you do it, you'll be surprised how much more aware of your face muscles you are—proof that you don't use them much in the normal course of a day.

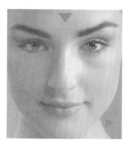

SMOOTHS the brow and tightens the jowl area.

1 Using your thumb and index finger together, gently pick up folds of skin all over your face, and gently squeeze then release them. This exercise stimulates the circulation and wakes up the face. Continue for one minute.

MAKE THE DIFFERENCE

Do this routine daily for seven days—and you'll notice a more youthful tone in your face at the end of the week.

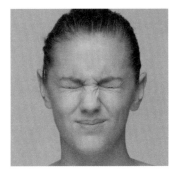

2 Make a really screwed-up face, hold it for three seconds, then slowly release your muscles. Repeat this exercise three times. This move tenses and relaxes all the facial muscles and works on areas that may not normally be well exercised.

3 With your mouth closed, pretend you are chewing something. Notice the direction in which you chew naturally, and do this exercise for about half a minute; then try to chew the other way. Don't overdo this movement, just chew slowly for about one minute in total. This exercise stretches the muscles of the jaw area and also the chin.

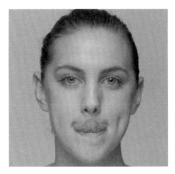

4 Stick your tongue out and try to touch the tip of your nose. Don't force this movement; go only as far as you can, then relax. This movement exercises the muscles under the chin area. Repeat three times.

5 With your lips closed, use your tongue to "brush" your teeth; this action creates a really interesting feeling, because the tongue is so sensitive. As well as increasing the production of saliva in your mouth, the movement of your tongue exercises muscles in the cheeks and chin. Continue for about one minute.

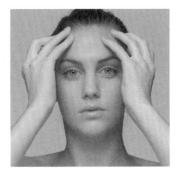

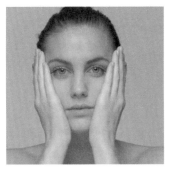

6 Using your fingertips, push the skin of your forehead up toward the hairline, then down toward the eyebrow line. This exercise makes you aware of how thin the layer of skin and muscle is over this area. Repeat three times.

7 Rub your hands together briskly, then place them over your face and feel the warmth beneath them. Breathe deeply several times.

53

Exercise your forehead

The forehead shows not only aging lines but also facial expressions caused by stress, such as frown marks. We often don't realize that our repetitive thoughts and stresses literally make their mark on our faces. These exercises will help release that stress and mitigate its effects on your face.

To prepare, sit comfortably on a hard-back chair, with your legs uncrossed and hands resting lightly in your lap. You may like to play some pleasant music while you work. Breathe easily and regularly throughout the exercise.

1 A short frown can be a good exercise; try it for three seconds and then slowly release. Feel the change in your facial muscles. When you are angry or intense, this muscle clenching is what happens to your face. Repeat three times, but without any stress!

2 Using your fingertips, push the skin of your forehead up toward the hairline, then down toward the eyebrow line. This exercise feels relaxing to do, and it makes you aware of how thin the layer of skin and muscle is over this bony area. Repeat three times.

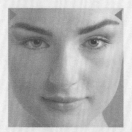

3 Place your fingers in your hair and rest the heels of your hands against the hairline. Tense your arms and hands and gently pull toward the back of your head, stretching the skin of the forehead. Hold for a few seconds, then relax. Repeat three times.

4 Place both hands over your forehead with your palms against the skin. Slowly squeeze out toward the sides of the forehead, imagining that you are "wiping away" tension. Repeat three times.

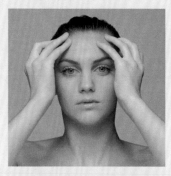

5 Use your fingertips to make tiny circular movements all along the very edge of your hairline. This exercise is amazingly relaxing and improves circulation to the area. It can also ease a headache. Continue for about one minute.

6 Close your eyes and focus on your forehead area. How does it feel now? Do you notice any feelings of tingling or warmth—these are signs of improved circulation and muscle tone. Do these exercises regularly and you will feel this all the time.

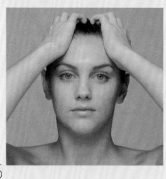

Work your cheeks & mouth

Signs of aging in the cheeks show up as slack muscles, which cause a drooping effect in the lower jaw area, perhaps with loose folds of skin. One of the best and simplest exercises is to chew some raw food, such as carrot or celery, at least once daily to exercise the muscles in the cheeks and around the mouth.

54

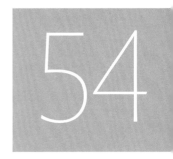

Sit comfortably in a hard-back chair, with your legs uncrossed and hands resting lightly in your lap. These exercises use sounds as well as face postures, so you might like to play some music to disguise the sounds you will make!

1 Take a deep breath and, as you exhale, make an exaggerated "aah" shape with your mouth, sounding the vowel at the same time. Do this slowly three times. Feel the muscles in your cheeks begin to stretch.

2 Breathe in, then exhale, and make an exaggerated "air" sound, feeling how the shape of your face changes as the vowel changes. Repeat three times.

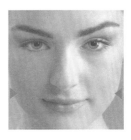

3 Breathe in, then exhale and make an exaggerated "ee" sound. As the sound changes, note that your face is now in a totally different shape and position. Repeat three times.

4 Breathe in, then exhale and make an exaggerated "or" sound; now your mouth is rounded and you can really feel the cheeks working hard. Repeat three times.

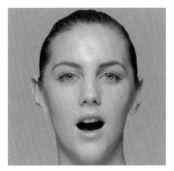

5 Breathe in, then exhale, and make an exaggerated "oo" sound. This position engages the ring of muscle around the mouth, the cheek area, and the muscles under the chin. Repeat three times.

6 Now slowly form all five sounds in turn—"aah," "air," "ee," "or," "oo—feeling your face working and changing as the sounds change. Repeat the whole sequence three times. Your face should now feel well exercised.

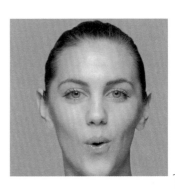

55 Firm up your chin

The chin area is connected to the neck and shoulders by a large area of powerful muscle called the sterno-cleido-mastoid. This extensive flap of muscle anchors in under the collarbone and connects to the chin as far up as behind the ear. The following exercises work this muscle in particular.

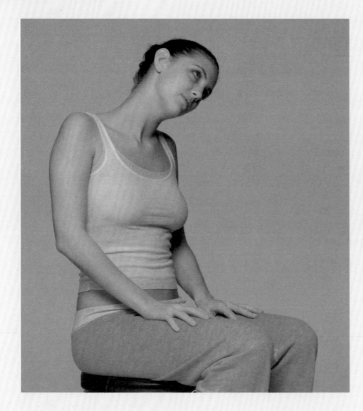

Sit comfortably on a stool with your back straight, your feet flat on the floor, and your hands resting in your lap.

1 Keeping your back straight and your shoulders still, tilt your head downward, comfortably.

2 Slowly roll your head toward your right shoulder, going only as far as you comfortably can.

3 Now gently tilt your head backward, being careful not to strain your neck, especially if you have problems in this area.

4 Finally, roll your head toward your left shoulder, before returning to the starting position to complete the circular movement.

Repeat the sequence once more, slowly, in the same direction, then twice more going in the opposite direction.

Exercise your jaw

Exercises for the jaw involve a very important joint called the temporomandibular joint (or TMJ). Some of the most important muscles in the face also connect into this area. Tension in your TMJ can cause toothache or headaches, and working it gently benefits the bony structure of the face as well as the muscles of the jaw.

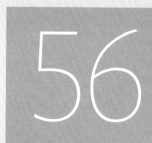

56

For this series of exercises, sit in a hard-back chair, with your legs uncrossed and your back straight. Don't overdo the movements, and if you feel any discomfort, stop straight away.

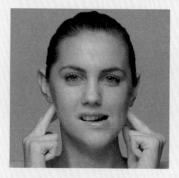

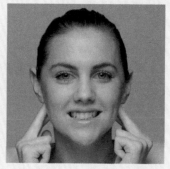

1 Place your fingers under your ears on either side of your face and locate the TMJ by opening and closing your mouth slightly three or four times.

2 Keep feeling with your fingers, and now exaggerate the opening and closing of your mouth by doing it more slowly and widely. You should really be able to feel the TMJ now. Repeat three or four times.

3 Still holding the TMJ area with your fingers, move your jaw from side to side, slowly and carefully. This feels quite different and you may find that one side is more mobile because you tend to chew in that direction. Repeat three or four times.

4 Now, clench your teeth, hold for three seconds, then release. Feel with your fingers how that affects the TMJ area and the cheeks as well as the jaw. Repeat slowly three times.

5 Now, using your fingers, massage the TMJ area using slow and careful little circles. Keep your mouth relaxed and slightly open. Continue for about half a minute.

6 Take a few deep breaths, and relax, noting any sensations in your jaw or face. Notice how different the area feels after these exercises. Doing this routine regularly will help to prevent grinding of the teeth resulting from jaw tension.

57

Try a cleansing facial for oily skin

Oily skin can make your face look prematurely old, causing unsightly shine and oxidation of the facial pores. If you have oily skin, keep it looking young with this great cleansing facial.

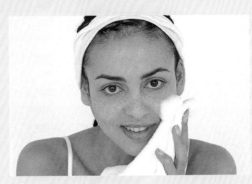

1 Cleanse. Apply a foaming (but soap-free) cleanser to your face, then, using a soft washcloth, gently rub the whole face in circular motions. This will break down oil and grime on the skin's surface, while the movement will exfoliate any dead cells.

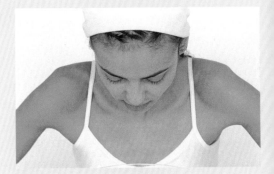

2 Steam your face. Boil some water and pour it into a large bowl. After the really hot steam has dispersed, lower your face over the bowl (keeping it at least ten inches off the water). Put a towel over your head and stay put for up to ten minutes.

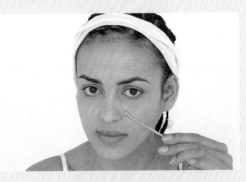

3 Use a blackhead extractor or wrap clean tissue around the tips of your fingers and gently apply pressure around the sides of the blackheads. Move the tissue regularly. When you've finished, apply a little witch hazel or tea tree oil.

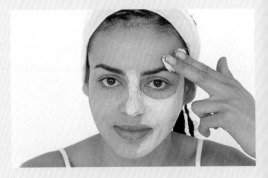

4 Apply a clay-base face mask. This will help draw out any more impurities and deep-cleanse the skin. If the mask makes your face sting, then it's too harsh for your skin: try our strawberry-base mask instead (see opposite).

TOP 5 TIPS FOR OILY SKIN

- Only cleanse twice a day. More often will trigger that panic response.

- If shine still slips through, blotting paper is great for mopping up excess oil.

- Make sure all your products—even your makeup—are oil free.

- Cut down on fast food. No, grease doesn't cause grease, but studies show that the iodine in fast food can contribute to acne on oily skin.

- If you get painful red acne, a little lavender oil dabbed on the skin will help reduce inflammation in minutes. In emergencies, whiteheads can be dried out with toothpaste.

YOUR 5 KEY PRODUCTS

- Foaming cleanser
- Oil-free moisturizer
- Clay mask
- Blotting papers
- Acne stick.

☞ MAKE YOUR OWN...

STRAWBERRY FACE MASK

A strawberry-base face mask will help cleanse oily skin without irritation. For an easy face mask blend together the following ingredients:

½ tsp lemon juice
1 egg white
1 tsp honey
½ cup strawberries

Leave the mask on cleansed skin for ten minutes and rinse off.

BELOW Strawberries have great astringent properties and will help cleanse oily skin without irritation. Try making a strawberry-base face mask.

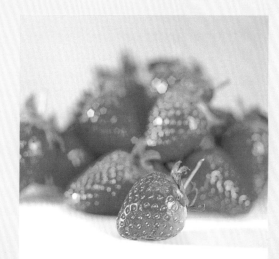

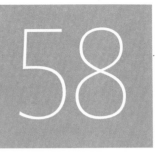

58

Hydrate dry skin with this moisture-boosting facial

Dry skin can make your face look old prematurely and can result in earlier wrinkles. Do this facial once or twice a week until moisture levels are boosted.

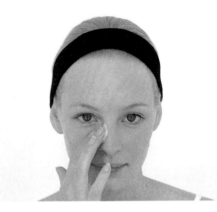

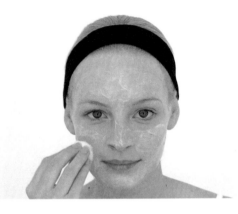

1 Exfoliate. Using your gentle facial scrub, rub the skin in a circular motion. Concentrate on areas like the nose and forehead. Some scrubs can dry the skin out, so rinse well.

2 Cleanse the skin with a milky cleanser. Doing this after the exfoliation will help remove any deep-down grime instead of just polishing the dead skin cells on the surface. Wipe it away with cotton balls: it's less absorbent than tissues and so will leave more protection on the skin.

3 Spritz or splash your skin. Toners are a no-no on dry skin because they will dehydrate it. Instead, freshen up your face with a spritz of facial mist or a splash of cool water. Absorb any excess afterward but don't completely dry the skin.

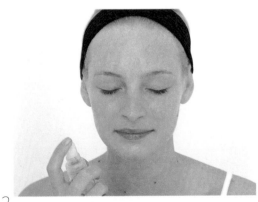

4 Now apply a hydrating mask. Look for emollient or humectant ingredients in these. Leave this for 10 to 15 minutes, then rinse off. Again, leave the face damp.

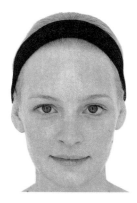

5 Apply your moisturizer. The best way to do this is by patting the skin with your fingers—this helps bring blood to the skin's surface, which will help hydrate it from within.

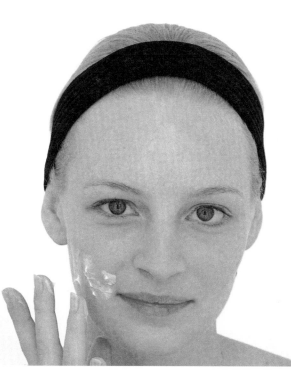

59

For combination skin, try this balancing facial

This once-a-week treat intensively tackles both the dry and oily areas of your skin. It will keep your face looking toned, taut, and—above all—youthful!

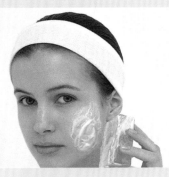

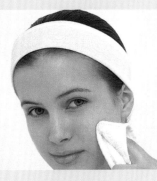

1 Cleanse your face using a moisturizing facial bar or a foaming cleanser. This will effectively target the oil on the greasy skin of the T zone, without removing any of the moisture from the dry skin on your cheeks.

2 Exfoliate to avoid flakes of dry skin clogging pores. Using a gentle facial scrub or a washcloth, rub the cheeks lightly. Go more intensely when tackling the greasy areas of the face to help loosen blackheads.

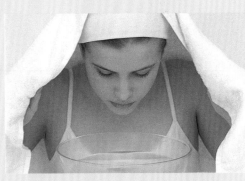

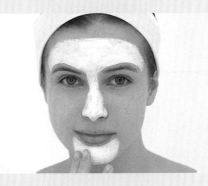

3 Boil a saucepan of water and pour some into a large bowl. Add four drops of rose water to the bowl. Lower your face over the bowl, keeping it ten inches off the water. Put a towel over your head and stay put for up to ten minutes.

4 Shop around for a hydrating moisture mask you apply to your cheeks and throat and a clay-base mask for the oily areas. Leave the masks on for ten minutes and rinse with tepid water before applying your normal light moisturizer.

TOP 5 TIPS FOR COMBINATION SKIN

- Don't scrub oily areas—this irritates the skin and increases oil production.

- Don't treat your whole face the same. Your T zone will require cleansing twice a day, while the cheeks only need doing once.

- After using pore strips, apply tea tree oil to your nose. It will reduce redness and cut bacteria levels in the pores.

- Avoid leave-in hair conditioners. Ingredients in these block the forehead's pores, making already greasy skin worse.

- Don't forget eye creams: You may need to avoid rich moisturizers on your cheeks, but you shouldn't skip them on the delicate skin around your eyes.

YOUR 5 KEY PRODUCTS

- Cleansing bars
- Pore strips
- Exfoliating scrub
- Oil-free moisturizer
- Eye cream.

BELOW Rose petals contain exactly the natural ingredients that both dry and oily skin needs for perfect balance and to look its best at all times.

☞ MAKE YOUR OWN...

ROSE-BASE FACE MASK

A rose-base mask is an excellent balancing treatment for combination skin. Use the following ingredients:

1 rose
1 tbsp rose water
1 tbsp plain yogurt
1 tbsp honey

Wash the rose petals in water. Soak for a few minutes and then crush them in a bowl. Add the rosewater, yogurt, and honey. Mix well and apply to the skin.

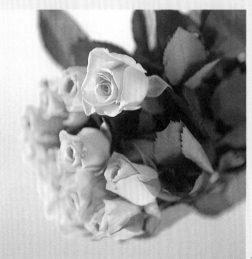

60

Relax with this calming facial for sensitive skin

Once a month, treat your skin to a facial designed to calm and stabilize. There aren't many steps here because the aim is to reduce your exposure to too many ingredients.

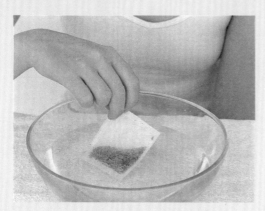

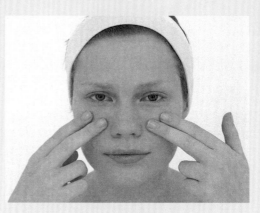

1 Camomile is incredibly calming, so for this session we're going to skip your cleanser and opt for a soothing camomile wash instead. Soak four camomile teabags in hot water. Once the water has cooled to warm, splash your face with this 20 to 30 times.

2 While your skin is still damp, stroke or tap the skin rapidly in downward motions. This helps drain away fluids and toxins under the skin's surface—and the fewer toxins there are in your system, the less chance there is of allergic reactions occurring.

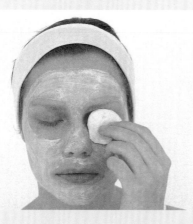

3 Apply a hydrating face mask from a hypoallergenic range, or try a soothing moisturizing mask. Because sensitive eyes can often feel red and itchy, give them a treat by applying some cotton balls soaked in the camomile mixture of Step 1. Relax for five to ten minutes, then wash off the mask with tepid water. Stroke a soft cloth gently across the face to remove any excess. Don't rub the skin—it will only make it redder. Finish off with a cooling gel moisturizer. For ultimate soothing power, put the gel in the refrigerator before you apply it.

TOP 5 TIPS FOR SENSITIVE SKIN

• Use products with fewer than ten ingredients to reduce the risk of coming across something you're allergic to.

• Wear sunscreen. Choose one that contains physical instead of chemical blocks such as titanium dioxide, and is less likely to cause an allergic reaction.

• Alternate products. The skin tends to become sensitized to things it encounters often. Find two different products and alternate every few weeks.

• Read labels. If you know you're allergic to a particular ingredient, avoid it.

• If you're really allergic, use only water and hydrocortisone cream for six months. Introduce gentle products one at a time.

YOUR 5 KEY PRODUCTS

• Facial wipes
• Eye makeup remover
• Light moisturizer
• Chemical-free sunscreen
• Hydrocortisone cream.

BELOW Oats and yogurt can help rehydrate and nourish irritated or damaged skin. Always buy the best and freshest ingredients that you can afford.

☞ MAKE YOUR OWN...

OAT AND YOGURT FACE MASK
This soothing mask helps reduce irritation. It's also great on sun-damaged skin. Use the following ingredients:

1 cup plain yogurt
¼ cup oats

Blend the yogurt and oats together. Mix well and apply to the skin for ten minutes. Rinse off with warm water.

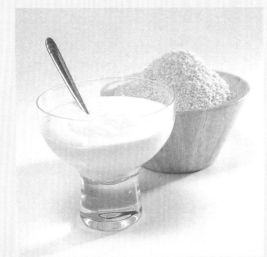

61

Treat yourself to a firming facial for maturing skin

This once-a-week facial hydrates intensely, but also uses massage techniques to boost circulation and tighten and firm the skin. It is a great boon to skin that has begun to age visibly.

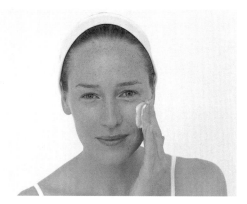

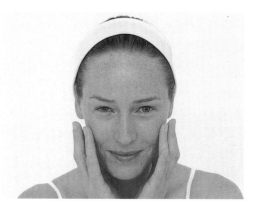

1 Cleanse the skin using a milky cleanser, applying it directly onto your face with your fingers. Let it sink in for a few seconds, then, using circular movements (always moving up the face), massage it in. Remove with cotton balls in the same fashion. This will increase circulation to the skin.

2 Starting at your chin, move around the edge of the jaw and face, lightly tapping the skin 10 to 20 times at points an inch apart. Do the same around the eyes. This will help boost circulation and reduce puffiness, creating a firmer look.

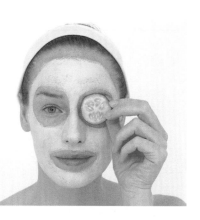

3 Apply an exfoliating mask. This will get rid of dead skin cells but is more hydrating than a facial scrub alone (try a peel-off cucumber mask). Apply tightening cucumber pads (or slices of the real thing) to your eyes and relax. Rinse off, finishing by splashing the face 10 to 20 times with cold water. This boosts circulation, ready for the treatments to come.

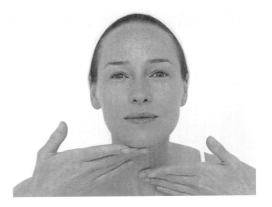

4 Apply a vitamin serum, again using upward stroking movements but this time from the neck. Slap the underside of your chin 20 times.

5 Finish with a thick coat of rich moisturizer. Let it soak in for five minutes, then remove any excess with cotton balls.

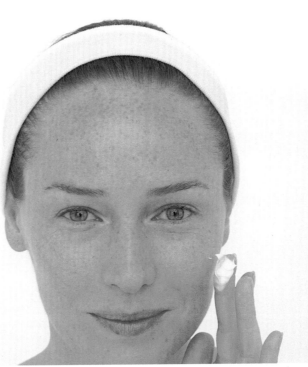

62

Release your tension

For face-lift purposes, a gentle head rub is a marvelous way to relax the whole head and face, improving circulation and easing stress. This sequence is easy to give to yourself; you can do it on dry hair or try it in the shower with shampoo. It will give you an invigorating start—or end—to the day!

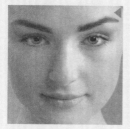

1 Place both hands in your hair on top of your head, and rest them there, breathing deeply. Feel the heat gather under your fingers—it's surprising how warm the top of the head is.

2 Move your hands in your hair slowly, making firm, circular massage movements all over the top, sides, and back of your skull. Use your thumbs and fingertips to get good pressure, stimulating the scalp and muscles over the skull.

3 Using the heels of your hands, massage slowly and deeply in the area just above your ears, making circles one way and then the other. Your cheek muscles actually connect in here.

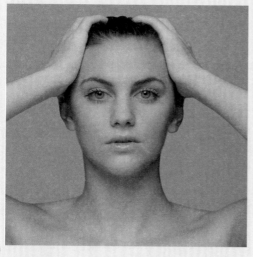

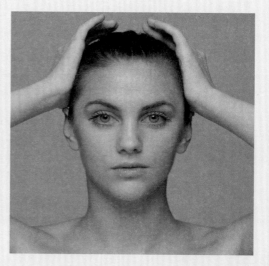

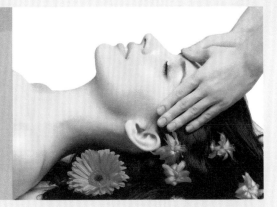

✳ TIP BOX

MASSAGE TO RELAX
In India, China, and the Far East, head massage is a part of everyday life. People of all ages exchange it with each other. As well as stimulating the scalp, head massage works on muscles that attach to the skull; these can contribute to headaches or migraines if they remain tense. Eastern head massage is marvelous as a nourishing and nurturing self-treatment. Relieving stress also has an important part to play in facial rejuvenation.

4 Bring the heels of your hands to your temples and repeat the same circular movements—these areas respond well to touch, and a lot of tension is stored here. You are improving muscle tone and circulation close to your eyes.

5 Use your thumbs to massage deeply at the base of the skull behind the ears; this action is wonderfully beneficial to the circulation of the neck and jaw area and helps to prevent migraine.

6 Finally, stroke your head from front to back, running your hands through your hair slowly. This feels very soothing and makes you feel that you are taking care of yourself. Repeat as often as you like—whatever makes you feel good.

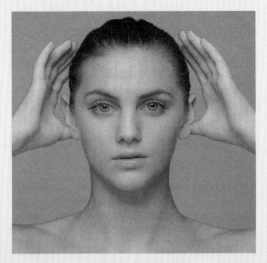

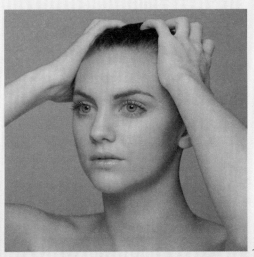

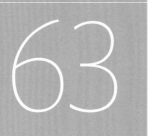

Enjoy a basic face massage

This exercise is a useful introduction to massage. Massage is a special form of touch that works specifically to increase blood flow to muscles, easing away toxins and releasing tension. In face massage work, you need to get used to working on small muscles with precise movements.

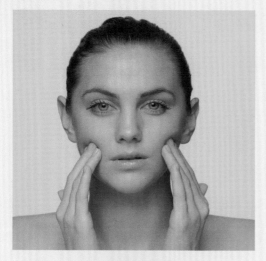

This simple massage uses the first and most basic massage movement—stroking. It involves the fingertips and palms of the hands. To massage comfortably, it is best to have short nails. For the massage, use one teaspoon of carrier oil, such as apricot kernel, to lubricate the skin.

1 **Stroking up from the chin** Start with your hands on either side of the face; with your palms and fingertips, stroke slowly up the sides of the face and up to the forehead, then glide back down again lightly. Repeat three times. The emphasis in the movement is pressure up the face, and then easing off.

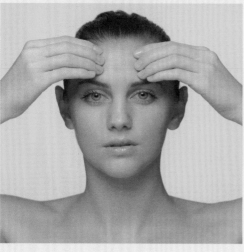

2 **Stroking out over the forehead** Place your fingertips together in the middle of your forehead, then press firmly and glide out to the sides; lift the fingers off, return to the starting pose, and repeat three times. This movement smooths out the forehead.

MORE BASIC MASSAGE TECHNIQUES

• Kneading the chin—make small kneading movements all the way along your jaw, up to your ears.

• Knuckling the cheeks—make your hands into loose fists and knuckle all around your cheekbones.

• Circling the forehead—use the heels of your hands to make large circles over your forehead.

• Tapping the face—energize your face by tapping lightly all over it with your fingertips.

3 **Stroking around the eyes** Using only a minimal amount of oil to ease the movement, place your fingertips at the sides of your eyes and stroke around the bony edge of the eye socket. Work up over the eyebrows, down the center of the nose, under the eyes, and back to the starting position. Repeat three times. This movement helps to improve eyestrain, and the oil will lubricate the skin around the eye area.

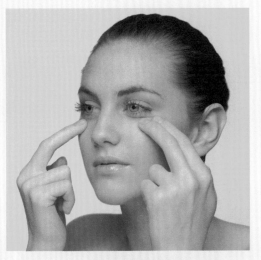

4 **Stroking under the cheekbones** Starting close to the nose, with your hands on the inner side of each cheek, make small circular pressures all the way out toward your ears. Give special attention to the area just under the ear (the location of the temporomandibular joint), then massage back toward the nose. Repeat the sequence three times. This movement tones the cheek muscles, which work hard every day.

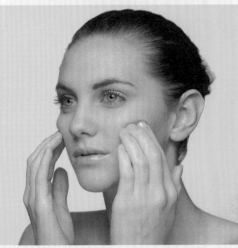

Get a glowing complexion

This deep circulation stimulating routine is especially good for mature skins that look dull or pale due to poor circulation. It gets the blood moving properly around the face and gives a glow to the complexion. Not only will this routine make your skin look younger, it will also give you an invigorating lift.

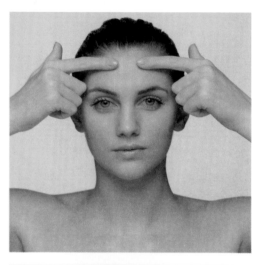

Before performing this routine, try a simple oatmeal scrub to gently exfoliate the skin surface. In a small bowl, place two tablespoons of fine oats, and add enough water to mix to a paste. Apply this mixture to your face with small circular movements, avoiding the eye area, and then remove with warm water and pat your skin dry.

For the blend, use one teaspoon of nourishing jojoba carrier oil with one drop of frankincense essential oil for cell renewal.

1 **Pressing across the forehead** Bring your index fingers together to meet in the middle of your forehead at your hairline. Make a line of pressures out toward the sides of the forehead. Then bring the fingertips back together, a little farther down, and make a second line of pressures out to the sides of the forehead. Continue until you reach eyebrow level. (Four lines of horizontal pressures are usually enough.)

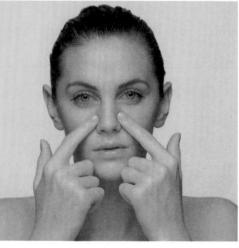

2 **Pressing down the sides of the nose** Bring the tips of your index fingers together between your eyebrows and stroke slowly down the sides of your nose, pressing firmly, to the level of your mouth. Lift your fingers off and repeat the movement three times. Sometimes this area can be a little tender, so be gentle.

3 **Stretching and lifting the cheeks** Using all your fingertips, with one hand on either side of your nose, stroke out over the cheeks to the sides of your face, stretching the skin under your hands, then release. Repeat this movement three times.

4 **Alternate stroking under the chin** Using one hand after the other, slowly and firmly stroke up the neck and under the chin in a series of sweeping movements. Keep the strokes firm and flowing. This stroke encourages good muscle tone in the chin and lower jaw area and is vital for lifting sagging skin.

Try a facial detox

This routine improves overly oily or blemish-prone skin with a combination of skin-cleansing ingredients and massage movements to encourage the drainage of toxins. It uses sweeping movements down the face to enhance detoxification via the lymphatic glands in the sides of the neck.

65

Before the massage, try a special facial steam to deep-cleanse the face. Pour four cups of almost boiling water into a heatproof glass bowl, and add two tablespoons of dried camomile flowers. Remove contact lenses, if wearing. Lean over the bowl with your head under a towel, and let the soothing steam bathe your face for ten minutes. Rinse your face afterward with warm water and pat dry.

For the blend, combine one teaspoon of jojoba carrier with one drop of cleansing lemon essential oil.

1 **Wide circles down the face** First, to apply the lemon-scented oil, make wide circular movements across your forehead, down your cheeks and nose to your chin. These strokes need to spread the oil over the whole surface of the face. Work from the middle of the face outward to encourage drainage.

2 **Small circles from the cheeks down** Working from under the eyes down to the chin, make a series of lines of small circular pressures, working outward in horizontal lines from the nose area to the sides of the face. You will probably find that four horizontal lines of pressures will be enough to travel from under your eyes to your chin.

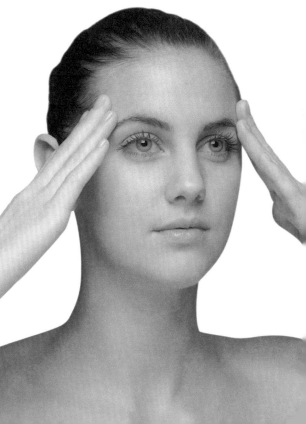

3 **Alternate cheek movement** With a hand on each cheek, make a series of large circles on alternate cheeks, moving the whole cheek area each time. Keep this stroke slow but the pressure firm. This movement exercises the muscles in the cheeks, chin, and jaw. Repeat several times, and feel how your whole face loosens up.

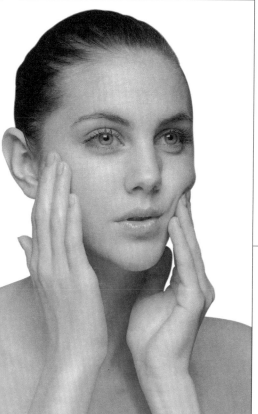

4 Sweeping strokes down the face Starting at your forehead, with fingertips meeting in the middle, stroke slowly all the way down the sides of your face to the chin and then sweep down to the neck. Bring the fingers back to the starting point and repeat the whole movement three more times. This movement encourages the drainage of toxins from the face.

Revive your complexion

This deep facial rejuvenation routine is a wonderful facial treat that is particularly suited to dry and mature skin types. It can be given once or twice a week to nourish and revive the complexion and tone the facial structure. It is one of the best routines for maintaining a youthful look for longer.

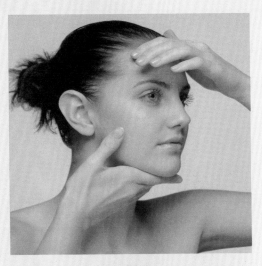

Before the massage, thoroughly cleanse and tone your skin. Soak a clean washcloth in tepid water combined with two drops of soothing lavender essential oil; wring out any excess water and place the hot washcloth over your face for a minute to gently hydrate and open your pores. For the blend, prepare two teaspoons of sweet almond oil with one drop of frankincense and one drop of mandarin essential oil stirred in to tone and revitalize your face.

1 **Cupping the face** With a little oil blend on your hands, cup one hand over your forehead and one under your chin. Hold for a few moments, relax, breathe deeply, and inhale the aroma of the blend. Gradually smooth the blend over the upper and lower halves of the face using your fingertips.

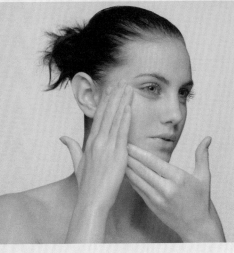

2 **Alternate stroking up the cheeks** Starting at chin level, make sweeping upward strokes on one cheek using both hands alternately, one following the other, then transfer across to the other side. This movement helps to improve circulation as well as toning the muscles of the cheek and chin area, increasing lift. It is also a very relaxing and soothing stroke.

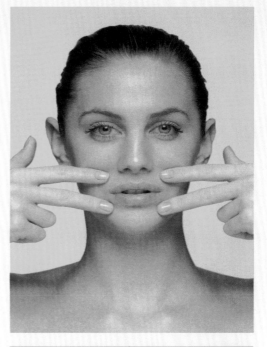

3 **Stretching around the mouth** Use your index and
middle fingers in a V shape placed around your
mouth. Slowly draw the fingers apart and out over
your cheeks; release, come back to the starting
position, and repeat three times. This movement helps
to massage the ring of muscle around the mouth and
ease out fine lines.

4 **Alternate upward strokes on the forehead** Using
the palms of your hands one after the other, stroke
firmly and slowly up the forehead using alternate
movements, one hand following the other. As well
as smoothing out lines, this move is also very soothing
for headaches or eyestrain. Repeat the movements
for two minutes.

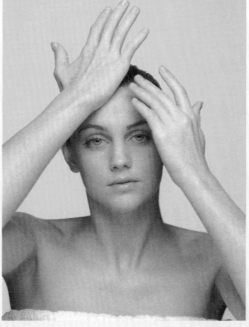

67

Reenergize your face with natural light

It might not seem very obvious, but your face needs plenty of light to look its best and remain fresh and healthy. Without regular exposure to daylight, your complexion will suffer.

SUNLIGHT—HARMFUL OR BENEFICIAL?

In our modern society, we find that we are spending much less time outside. This is because our work and living habits take us from one internal environment to another, all full of recycled air and artificial light. Our answer to this kind of existence is to jet off for a short period of time each year to places where the sun is very powerful, and then proceed to expose all our skin to that intensity of sunlight. This practice is not good for the skin and encourages damage through burning, as well as cellular damage and premature aging, which is why using powerful sunscreens is important when on vacation.

SEASONAL AFFECTIVE DISORDER

However, full-spectrum light—daylight, especially when the sun is at its peak, around midday—is actually scientifically proven to be vital to overall health. People who have SAD (Seasonal Affective Disorder) are depressed and low because of light deprivation. Studies have shown that going out for a walk, even for just ten minutes each lunchtime, exposes you to enough full-spectrum daylight to counter feelings of depression, low energy, or even premenstrual syndrome. Light

acts on the pineal gland in your skull, which is linked to the pituitary gland that controls the balance of hormones in the body.

STRONG LIGHT IN MODERATION

Moderate exposure to sunlight at the latitude where you normally live is actually beneficial to your skin, whatever your age; it encourages a healthy glow and helps to heal blemishes, as well as assisting the body to manufacture vitamin D, which you need for bone formation and healthy joints. Obviously we expose our skin less in the colder months, and as the seasons warm up, we can slowly accustom our skin to the sun. Well-established spas and health farms everywhere recommend spending regular time in strong light on a daily basis.

TEN-MINUTE TREAT

So give yourself a free ten-minute treat of light each day for health, vitality, and a radiant skin. It's easy to do, fits in with any schedule, and helps you to stay positive, even in the long winter months. It may be a very simple thing to do, but you will be making an important contribution to improving your health and well-being.

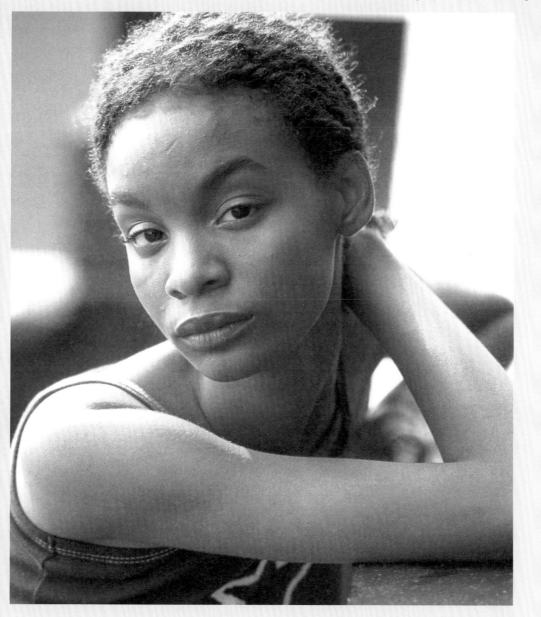

Relax before bed

Poor-quality sleep prevents our self-regenerating mechanisms from repairing and restoring us at cellular level, resulting in a tired and dull complexion. However, sleeping difficulties can be helped by adopting a simple relaxing routine at the end of the day, designed to help you unwind.

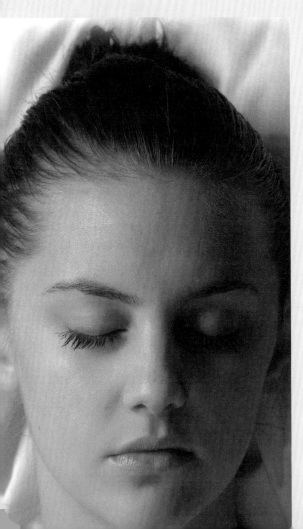

Before performing this presleep routine, have a relaxing warm bath or shower, and a warm drink, such as a herbal tea made with camomile or lime flower, or a simple mug of warm milk with a sprinkle of nutmeg on top. Get yourself comfortable in bed, with only a very dim light on, and no music or television to distract you. Pause between each step and breathe easily for a moment before continuing.

1 Lie on your back with a low pillow under your head. Close your eyes and breathe regularly and evenly.

2 Start by tensing all the muscles in your legs and feet, hold this position for a few moments, then slowly release.

3 Tense your arms and clench your hands into fists, hold this position for a few minutes, then slowly release.

4 Tense the muscles in your abdomen for a few moments, then slowly release.

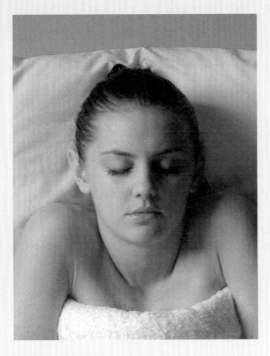

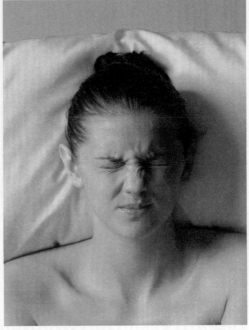

5 Tense your shoulders and hunch them up toward your ears, hold this position for a few moments, then slowly release.

6 Finally, screw your face up into a grimace, hold this position for a few moments, then slowly release.

When you have finished, lie still and simply breathe, noticing how your body feels. You may find that you fall asleep before the end, which is, of course, the ideal end to a presleep routine! Relaxed muscles will help you to obtain good-quality sleep and all the nourishment that brings.

04

Natural beauty

Your body is your temple, as the old saying goes, and it needs a little worship to remain feeling its best and most youthful. This chapter is full of tips on how to keep your skin, complexion, hands, feet, and hair in tip-top condition without resorting to aging cosmetics. It shows you how to slow the natural aging process while pampering yourself and building a little luxury into your life. Stay young and healthy the natural way.

Introduction

No matter what age you are, you can always make the most of what you have. Of course, there is a plethora of cosmetics and synthetic treatments available to help you do this, but it is so much healthier and more gratifying to care for your body and looks the natural way. It will keep you looking younger, too.

NATURAL IS BEST

The chances are that you have used makeup for a large part of your adult life. It might have made you look and feel better about yourself, but if it was based on synthetic chemicals and materials, as most mainstream cosmetics are, then it could have taken a toll on your looks and had a negative influence on the natural aging process of your skin. If this is the case, the good news is that it is never too late to change the way you go about making yourself look your best. For centuries, makeup preparations have been made from natural ingredients that are beneficial to your skin and body; in recent years these have made a substantial comeback to popularity and are now more widely available than ever before. Why not try some of these instead of the synthetic cosmetics you have used up to now? By the same token, there are numerous natural treatments and therapies, which, if undertaken regularly, can hold back the march of time on your body.

PAMPERING FOR PRESERVATION

In this chapter, we offer you a series of delectable treatments and therapies, from body scrubs made from natural ingredients to at-home hydrotherapy and enticing pick-me-ups for your hair, hands, feet, and legs. Follow these few basic tips as well and start keeping yourself young the natural way:

- Surprise yourself with sugar—sugar contains glycolic acid, an alpha hydroxy acid that effectively diminishes and prevents wrinkles. Glycolic acid rapidly detaches dead and damaged skin cells that accumulate on the face and create fine lines and deep creases. Use sugar in your skin applications and start to see the benefits.
- Get into olive oil—olive oil combined with vitamin E oil makes an intensive nighttime antiaging treatment. Olive oil has been used for centuries to preserve youthful and beautiful skin. It contains cleansing as well as moisturizing properties while vitamin E regenerates and repairs skin cells.
- Advantages of avocado—avocado has more protein and natural oils than any other fruit. It has been used as a natural beauty tool for generations, and can be used as an antiaging facial mask.

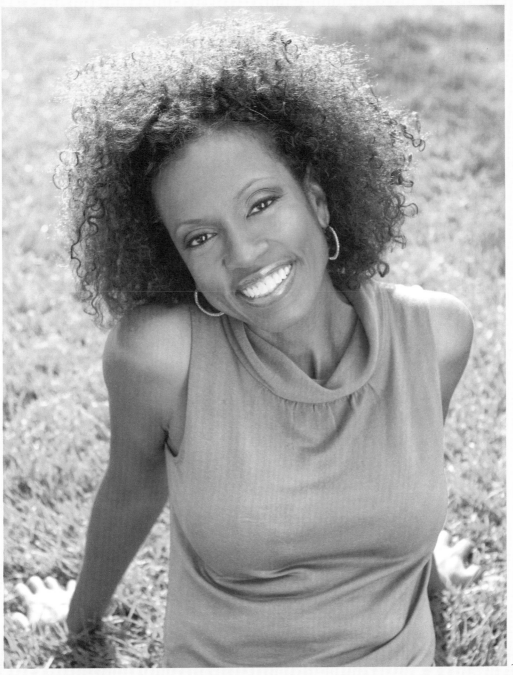

69

Brush away dry skin

Dry skin brushing is a great way to give your circulation a boost and improve the look of your skin. This age-fighting treatment is especially effective at getting rid of bumpy skin on the backs of your arms and at tackling the appearance of cellulite. An essential part of your summer beauty armory!

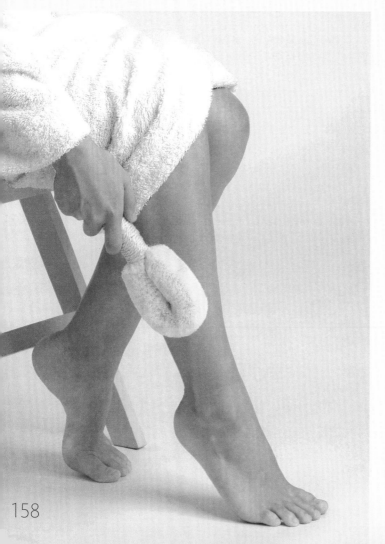

WHEN TO DO IT
The best time to do it is before you have a shower. You'll need a high-quality dry skin brush with soft bristles.

HOW TO DO IT
Start at the feet and, using a light but firm touch, start to sweep the brush in small circular motions over the skin. Move over the toes and up the legs, toward the hips. Next, start at the fingertips and continue up toward the heart. Go gently over delicate areas, such as the neck.

FINISHING OFF
When you've finished, get in the shower and lather yourself with a moisturizing shower gel. Your complexion should be left with a pink, healthy glow.

LEFT Brushing yourself in this way every other day or so is good for your circulation as well as your skin.

Make a toning body scrub

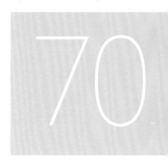

The key to soft, smooth skin is regular exfoliation. It helps to get rid of dead skin cells, so your complexion will appear more radiant. It's also the perfect way to prepare for self-tanning, because it will ensure a more even color. Your skin will also be primed to absorb all the nourishing ingredients in your moisturizer.

WHAT YOU WILL NEED
For this great exfoliating scrub mixture, you will need finely ground sea salt and a bottle of grapefruit-base essential oil. Both ingredients should be readily available from your local health store or drugstore.

1 Place three tablespoons of fine sea salt in a small bowl; add six drops of grapefruit essential oil, and stir them in thoroughly. Get in the shower, but do not turn the water on yet.

2 Take a handful of the mixture and rub it briskly all over your body, paying special attention to your thighs and stomach.

3 Rinse the mixture off the skin thoroughly. Grapefruit is cleansing and detoxifying, and the sea salt is an excellent exfoliator, removing loose, dead cells, and leaving the skin glowing and ready for moisturizing.

RIGHT This simple therapy will give your skin a revivifying treat.

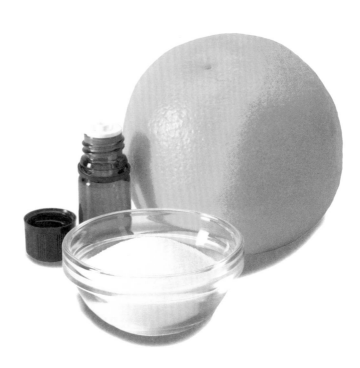

71

Scrub your skin soft

This unperfumed shower gel gives a lathering base; peppermint and rosemary are cleansing and refreshing herbs; sea salt provides the exfoliation; and the olive oil adds a skin-nourishing touch to the body scrub. For two treatments, you need four tablespoons of unperfumed shower gel.

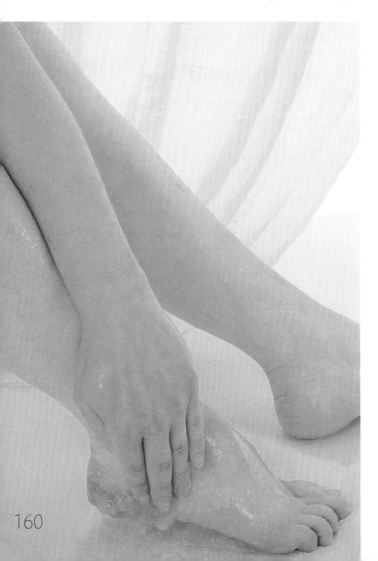

1 Pour this into a small dish and add two tablespoons of very finely chopped peppermint and rosemary leaves, one tablespoon of fine sea salt, and one tablespoon of extra-virgin olive oil.

2 Stir these ingredients together well. Rub over the body, especially over problem areas so you are energized and invigorated.

This method works well if you get in the shower and let warm water run over the skin before working up the body scrub to a lather. Change the temperature to much cooler, letting the jets pummel your body. Change back to warm and apply more of the body scrub and work into the skin. Rinse off and towel yourself dry.

LEFT This treatment is particularly good for smoothing and softening hard and "dead" areas of skin on the body, like that around your heels.

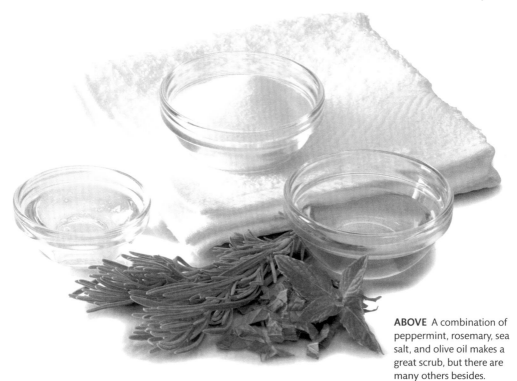

ABOVE A combination of peppermint, rosemary, sea salt, and olive oil makes a great scrub, but there are many others besides.

TOP FIVE EXFOLIATING SCRUB COMBINATIONS

Here are some other exfoliating scrub combinations for you to try.

1 Finely crushed apricot seeds, mango, and almonds makes a great, lightly scented exfoliating scrub that your skin will cherish.

2 Try mixing a lush recipe of raspberry, almond, and kiwi that will gently exfoliate skin while lightly moisturizing it.

3 When your feet need a pick-me-up, try a soothing mixture of natural sugar crystals, vitamins A, C, E, pro-vitamin B5, olive oil, and tea tree oil.

4 Try taking a hot bath in a combination of exfoliating margarita extract and sea salt that kisses you with a light scent. This oil-free mixture relies on natural extracts to smooth and moisturize skin.

5 A good combination for a soothing and warming winter body scrub is a mixture of grape seed oil, rose hip oil, sea salt, green tea oil, kelp, vitamin C, vitamin E, and kiwi.

72

Improve your skin texture

Hydrotherapy is frequently offered in spas as an invigorating treatment that can help to improve the appearance and texture of the skin by toning, tightening, and stimulating the lymphatic system. You can try this hot and cold hydrotherapy method in the comfort of your own bathroom.

First, get in the shower and let the water run comfortably warm; use a little shower cream to lather up on the skin. Then change the temperature of the water to run much cooler, letting the jets pummel your body, particularly your chest, stomach, buttocks, and thighs. This is particularly effective if you have a powerful shower.

Change the temperature back to warm again, and this time massage in some of the grapefruit and sea salt body scrub described on page 159, using a cellulite massager to really work it into the skin.

Finally, rinse off all the scrub and towel yourself dry. You should feel invigorated and refreshed, with soft, glowing skin.

BELOW You don't need to confine at-home hydrotherapy to the shower—why not try it in your bathtub, as well? If you have a jacuzzi feature in your tub, so much the better. The whole point is to have a little relaxing "you" time in soothing hot water.

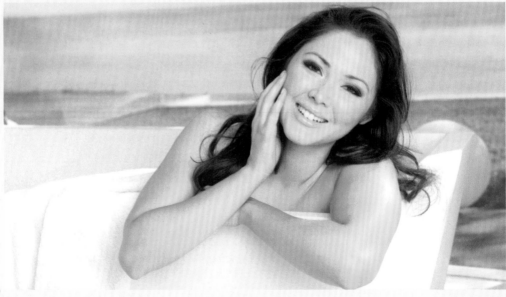

LEFT Turn the phone off, unplug the television and radio, get in the shower or bathtub, and relax. Make sure you have a lot of fluffy, freshly laundered towels to climb into afterward!

✳ **TIP BOX**

WATER FOR HEALTH
Baths and showers can also be used to treat a number of health problems. Hot baths are used to ease joint pain, constipation, and respiratory ailments, and cold baths relieve fever and fatigue.

73

Moisturize your skin

In hot weather, skin can easily become dehydrated, making it dry and less youthful-looking. To get it back to its plump, dewy best, you need to make sure you keep it well moisturized. Here we show you the best ways to rejuvenate your dry skin—the natural way.

DRINK A LOT OF WATER AND MOISTURIZE

Drinking a lot of water will help keep your skin looking young, because it hydrates from within. Of course, drinking water is always good for you in a lot of ways, so you can never really have enough (see pages 20–21). You can also combat the drying effects of the sun with a good moisturizing lotion or cream. Use it as a base before you apply your sunscreen; this will help it sink more easily into the skin, so you'll get a more even coverage (see illustration opposite).

ANTIAGING AGENTS

Look for a moisturizing lotion that contains antiaging antioxidants, such as vitamins A, C, and E, as well as nourishing oils—score extra beauty points if you find one with added SPF (sun protection factor). Basic baby oil is also a great moisturizer—but don't ever be tempted to use it as a replacement for sunscreen, because it will not offer you the same protection and will actually assist the burning process. You will always need to apply at least an SPF15 (if you have darker skin that tans easily) or up to SPF30 (if you are fair-skinned), in order to protect yourself from the skin-damaging effects of UV rays.

APPLYING YOUR MOISTURIZER

When you apply your moisturizer, start from your toes and work upward toward your chest and shoulders—and don't forget your neck. Gently massage it in using a firm touch, concentrating on areas that are typically prone to dryness, such as elbows, knees, and feet. Use your usual face cream, then apply sunscreen over the top. Try the nourishing aromatherapy blend described on the opposite page for a real skin treat.

* **TIP BOX**

SHEA BUTTER
Used in Africa for centuries and made from the nuts of the karite tree, shea butter is rich in natural vitamins that promote healthy skin and cell repair. It is now widely used in the beauty industry.

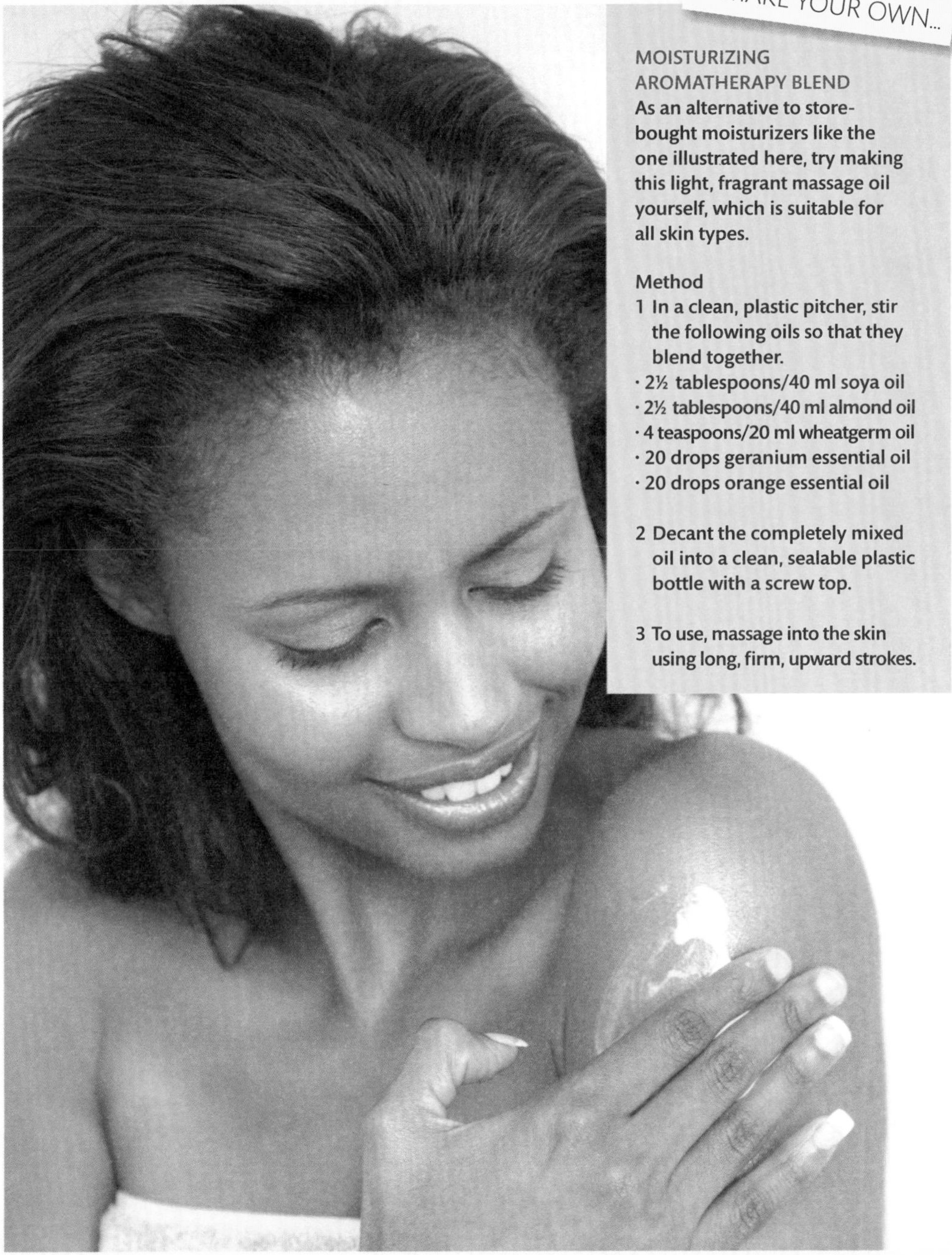

☞ MAKE YOUR OWN...

MOISTURIZING
AROMATHERAPY BLEND
As an alternative to store-bought moisturizers like the one illustrated here, try making this light, fragrant massage oil yourself, which is suitable for all skin types.

Method
1 In a clean, plastic pitcher, stir the following oils so that they blend together.
· 2½ tablespoons/40 ml soya oil
· 2½ tablespoons/40 ml almond oil
· 4 teaspoons/20 ml wheatgerm oil
· 20 drops geranium essential oil
· 20 drops orange essential oil

2 Decant the completely mixed oil into a clean, sealable plastic bottle with a screw top.

3 To use, massage into the skin using long, firm, upward strokes.

74

Exfoliate your face and body

Having silky smooth skin all over is an essential part of looking and feeling younger, especially if you are planning on having much of it on general display! If you are someone who enjoys swimming at your local pool or visiting the ocean, then carefully shaved and exfoliated skin is an absolute must.

BELOW Be careful not to nick yourself when you are shaving with either a disposable or electric razor. You can mitigate the problem by applying a little gel to your skin before you begin.

DE-FUZZ

Shaving is by far the quickest and cheapest way to de-fuzz your body. It's best to use a gel or foam, so the razor glides over your skin, making nips and cuts less likely. You should shave in the opposite direction from that in which your hair grows to get as close a shave as possible. You'll be silky smooth for a few days before you'll have to tackle regrowth, so remember to pack some disposable razors in your suitcase.

Sugaring is similar to waxing, although it's thought to be less painful because the sugar mixture sticks only to the hair, as opposed to the skin. It's made of natural ingredients and, while you can buy it premade in the stores, you can also make it yourself at home. Simply cook two cups of regular white sugar with a cup of water and a cup of lemon juice on the stove until the mixture forms a stiff paste. Dust the area of skin you want to de-fuzz with talcum powder, then apply the mixture with a spatula. Apply a piece of cloth or paper towels onto the mixture, then quickly pull it away in the opposite direction of hair growth, taking the hairs with it. The results should last for up to one week.

Waxing is the most effective, but arguably the most painful, way to get rid of body hair. You can buy prepared waxing strips in most drugstores, or pots of liquid wax, which you warm to melt before you use it. Waxing pulls hair out by the root—it's what causes the pain—and is carried out in the same way as sugaring.

Plucking is ideal for eyebrows and coarse hairs growing in inconspicuous places. If you want to tidy up your eyebrows, do so after a warm bath, because the steam opens up the skin's pores, making the process less painful. Use a magnifying mirror if you have one, and stretch out skin underneath the hairs with one hand, using the other to hold the tweezers and to pluck.

BE A REAL SMOOTHIE

Your face needs exfoliating too, but many body scrubs are too harsh to use on the delicate skin on your face. Try this recipe for a gentle almond, honey, and lemon facial scrub that can be used on even the most sensitive of skins. Ground almonds remove dead cells and smooth the skin, while honey is hydrating and lemon juice tones the pores.

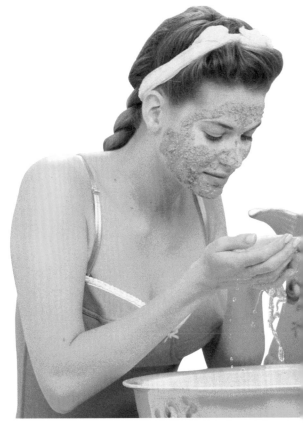

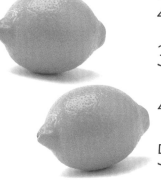

1 Place two tablespoons of ground almonds in a saucer. If you are allergic to nuts, substitute fine oats instead.

2 Add two tablespoons of good-quality honey and two tablespoons of lemon juice.

3 Mix all the ingredients together, then apply to the face in small circular movements.

4 Leave on for 15 minutes, then massage into the skin once more using warm water.

5 Rinse thoroughly and finish by applying a nourishing moisturizer or serum.

ABOVE When applying this gentle exfoliating mixture, use plenty of warm water in addition to make the impact on your facial skin as gentle as possible.

75

Tighten and tone your face

Many women swear by using a toner as part of their morning and evening beauty routine for soft and glowing skin. Toning lotions are designed to get rid of traces of make-up and tone and tighten pores, making them less visible. Try this recipe for a freshening melissa herbal toning lotion.

TIGHTEN AND TONE
Use this treatment after cleansing, but before moisturizing:

1 Prepare a melissa infusion by putting two tablespoons of chopped fresh melissa leaves in a small heatproof bowl.

2 Pour over ¾ cup of boiling water and let steep for 15 minutes. Strain, then refrigerate.

3 Apply the infusion to the skin with a cotton ball. Your skin should feel fresh and clean.

* **TIP BOX**

NATURAL ASTRINGENTS
Lemon juice, pureed peach juice, tomato juice, aloe vera, and the residue of pureed cucumbers are all excellent antiaging natural astringents that you could try as toners for your facial skin.

RIGHT & OPPOSITE
This gentle toning balm is made from melissa, but there are a lot of other natural alternatives to choose from as well.

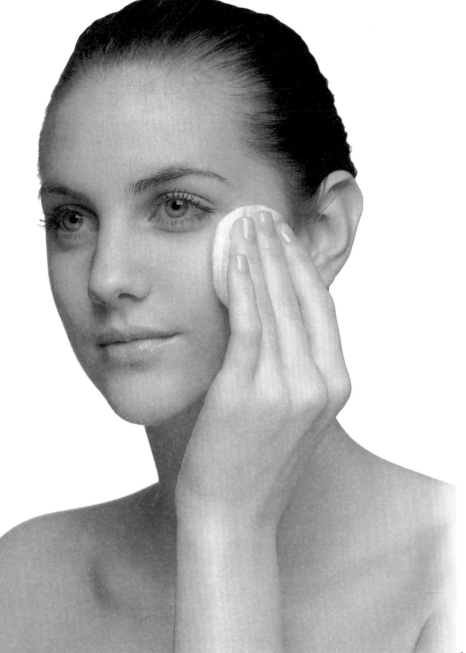

76

Purify your complexion

Your face has to put up with a lot. With the exception of your hands, it is consistently the most exposed part of your body, so it can fall prey to the vagaries of the weather, pollution, and home and office heating—any number of factors. This can mean clogged pores and facial blemishes. Here is how to avoid them.

This facial steam will help get rid of pore-clogging dirt and grime, and leave your skin squeaky clean. Simply follow the instructions below.

CAMOMILE AND MELISSA FACIAL STEAM

Steam opens up your pores and eliminates impurities, while melissa and camomile are extremely soothing to the skin.

1 Wash and chop a handful of fresh melissa leaves and camomile flowers.

2 Pour almost-boiling water into a medium heatproof bowl until it is half full.

3 Scatter the herbs on the surface of the water, then lean over the bowl with your face in the steam and your head under a towel. Stay under the towel for about 15 minutes, then wipe your face with a damp cloth and pat it dry.

RIGHT You can keep your skin looking as youthful as possible by putting in the groundwork once every week or so with a facial steam bath.

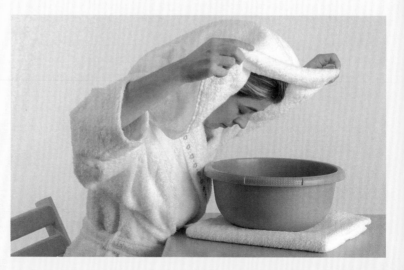

RIGHT A natural superfood packed full of vital nutrients and goodness, avocado combines well with other ingredients.

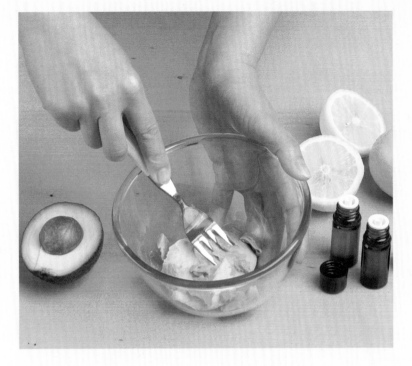

☞ MAKE YOUR OWN...

AVOCADO, CYPRESS, AND LAVENDER NOURISHING MASK
Avocado is full of vitamins A, D, and E, which nourish and protect the skin. Lemon juice and cypress oil tone the pores, and lavender acts as a soother.

1 In a small bowl, mash the flesh of half a ripe avocado.

2 Add one teaspoon of lemon juice, then two drops of cypress and three drops of lavender essential oils.

3 Apply the rich green paste all over the face, avoiding the eye area.

4 Leave on for 15 minutes, then wash off with tepid water and pat the skin dry.

77

Beautify your hands

After your face, your hands probably say more about you than any other part of your body. Unfortunately, hands that have been neglected in the beauty stakes are often the first thing to give your age away. Make sure yours are well and truly pampered with these natural recipes.

BELOW Ylang-ylang is a real oriental treat, whose gentle aroma will transport you mentally as well as physically as you treat your hands.

YLANG-YLANG WARM OIL HAND SOAK

Ylang-ylang is a skin-conditioning essential oil that has a lovely exotic floral aroma. This recipe will make enough oil to use on two pairs of hands. You can save any leftovers for a second application if desired—simply rewarm before use.

1 Pour enough almost boiling water to fill a medium heatproof bowl half way.

2 Pour four teaspoons of apricot kernel carrier into a smaller heatproof bowl and add four drops of ylang-ylang essential oil.

3 Stand the small dish in the larger bowl of hot water to warm the oil.

4 Once it has been heated through, lift the small dish out of the bowl and soak each hand in the warm oil for around five minutes. Wipe off any excess with a damp paper towel.

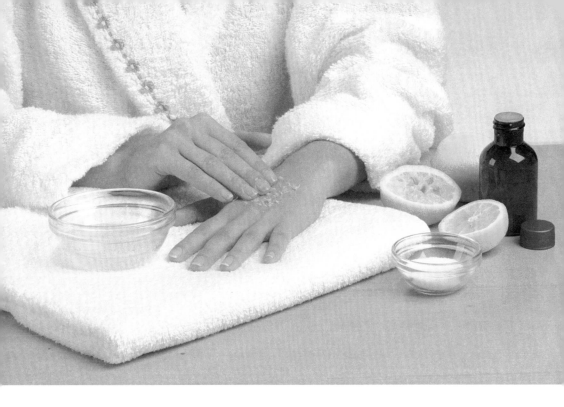

SUGAR AND LEMON EXFOLIATING SCRUB

This smells good enough to eat. Sugar granules gently exfoliate the skin while lemon tones and cleanses, and apricot oil helps soothe and nourish. This recipe should be enough to use on two pairs of hands—so you can treat a friend, also.

ABOVE This quietly decadent hand treatment will tone and refresh the skin of your hands as well as nourishing it thoroughly all over.

1 Put two tablespoons of granulated sugar in a small glass bowl.

2 Add the rind of one organic lemon and one tablespoon of lemon juice, plus two tablespoons of apricot kernel carrier oil. Stir together.

3 Apply a small amount of the mixture and work it gently into the hands, including all the fingers. Wipe off any excess with a damp paper towel.

78

Freshen up your feet

Smelly feet are a common problem in the summer months. It happens because the sweat glands are working in overdrive to try and cool the feet down (through sweating), but wearing shoes means that the skin cannot breathe properly and there is nowhere for the sweat to go.

The feet become warm and moist, creating an ideal environment for bacteria to thrive, and it is this that actually produces the odor. Sticking to open-toed shoes or sandals will help keep feet fresh, but if yours are still pungent, use these freshening recipes.

OLIVE OIL AND LAVENDER FOOT SCRUB

The olive oil in this recipe is supremely nourishing and great for dry skin, while the lavender helps to refresh and soothe the skin.

1 Pour six tablespoons of extra-virgin olive oil into a small bowl.

2 Add two teaspoons of fine sea salt—which makes an excellent exfoliator—and stir thoroughly into the olive oil.

3 Add 20 drops of lavender essential oil and stir to mix thoroughly.

4 Rest your feet on paper towels on top of a towel. Then carefully apply the scrub to one foot at a time, using small circular movements all over the foot, concentrating especially on any dry areas, such as the heels.

5 After massaging in the scrub for ten minutes, use the paper towels to wipe off any excess.

6 Repeat the massage with the other foot, again wiping off excess scrub at the end.

ROSEMARY HERBAL FOOT SOAK

As the rosemary leaves steep into the liquid, they will gently deodorize and tone the skin, helping to banish odor. For an extra-softening boost, add six tablespoons of whole milk to the water.

1 Fill a large plastic bowl halfway with warm water. It should be big enough to soak both your feet at once.

2 Add a handful of washed and chopped fresh rosemary leaves, and place your feet in the bowl. Add the whole milk if desired.

3 Let the feet soak for 15 minutes; if you have very dry heels, rub a pumice stone gently on the hard skin to smooth it.

4 Lift your feet out of the bowl and place onto a towel to dry thoroughly.

79

Foot and leg massage

A leg and foot massage can be incredibly relaxing. Not only will it help to minimize stiffness after exercise, but it will also encourage toxins out of the muscles, helping them work more effectively. Use this stimulating aromatherapy blend as a massage oil to encourage detoxification.

CYPRESS, LEMON, AND JUNIPER AROMATHERAPY BLEND

This makes enough to use on two pairs of legs—so you can save and reuse or treat a friend. Cypress tones the circulation while lemon and juniper encourage the elimination of toxins.

BELOW Treat your feet to a little bit of luxury with this toning and revivifying blend.

1 Pour four teaspoons of sweet almond oil into a small dish.

2 Add three drops of cypress oil, four drops of lemon oil, and three drops of juniper essential oil, and stir together. Use as needed.

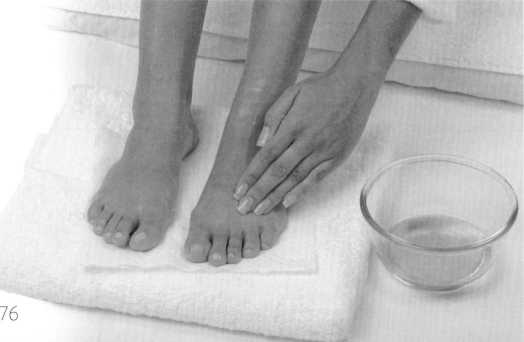

FOOT AND LEG MASSAGE

You need to enroll a willing friend to help you with this. Ask them to follow these instructions:

1 Set up the massage with your partner lying face down on the floor on a comfortable mat or futon covered with towels. Rest her head on a pillow and keep the upper part of the body covered and warm while you work on the legs. Kneel by your partner's feet or by the calves on whichever side feels most comfortable to you.

2 Stroke one teaspoon of the blend up both legs at the same time, starting from the feet and passing over the ankles, up the calves and thighs, to just below the buttocks. Spread the oil well, and repeat these strokes several times; apply more pressure up the leg and ease off as you come down.

3 Use the heels of your hands to apply slow, firm, circular pressure all over the soles of the feet and then over the calves. This soothing movement works all the main muscle groups.

4 Continue up the legs, using the heels of your hands to apply slow, firm pressure over the backs of the thighs. Be sensitive to your partner and check that the massage is comfortable for her.

5 Starting above the knees, make vertical lines of individual thumb pressure up toward the buttocks; press for a few moments, then move up a few inches and press again. Begin on the outsides of the thighs and work inward.

6 Repeat the strokes in step one, using long sweeps up the backs of both legs, with more pressure going up than coming down. Slow down the strokes and ease off to finish.

ABOVE RIGHT Use the blend described on the opposite page throughout this soothing massage.

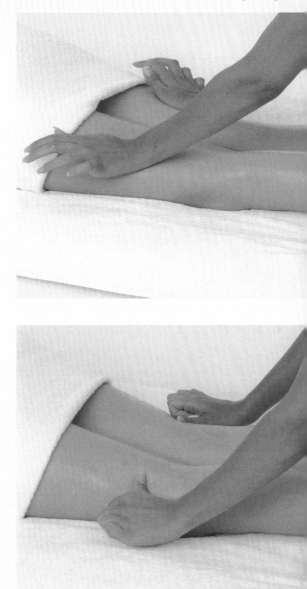

ABOVE Be careful to apply only gentle pressure and make sure that your friend is comfortable.

177

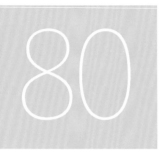

80

Manicures and pedicures

Well-manicured hands and feet will add the finishing touch to your healthy, youthful look. Well-cared-for nails make you appear more polished—literally!—and a bit of color will look great wherever you go. Vibrant reds, pinks, and oranges all look good and will brighten you up, so be adventurous.

EASY MANICURE AND PEDICURE

1 Massage a blob of moisturizing lotion into your hands and wipe any excess off your nails with a tissue.

2 Trim your nails with a pair of nail scissors so that they are all the same length.

3 Get rid of any rough edges with a nail file—aim for a classic oval shape.

4 Apply a base coat of clear nail polish—this will stop the colored polish from staining them. Let dry.

5 Apply the colored polish. For a streak-free finish, start by painting a line down the center of the nail, going from the nail bed to the tip of the nail. Then add more polish in the same way either side until the whole nail is evenly covered. Let dry, then add a second coat.

6 Add a clear top coat of varnish. It will help the color last longer and stop it from chipping. Remember to take the varnish and a nail file with you when you go out to top up the color if needed.

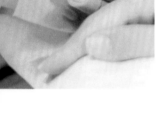

ABOVE A manicure won't take as long as you might think and can be a surprisingly effective aid to your bid to look younger.

OPPOSITE The best time to work on your toenails is directly after a bath, when they are at their softest and most pliant.

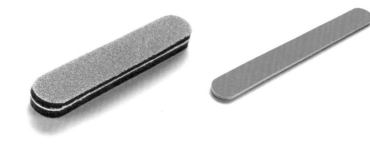

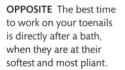

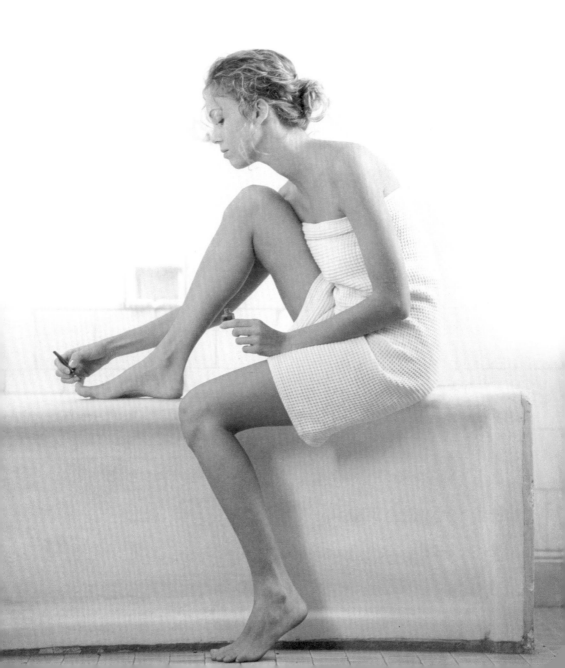

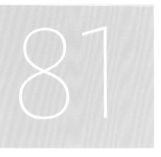

81 Invigorate your hair

If you spend a lot of time outdoors, especially in summer, the sun's rays can be incredibly drying to the hair. In order to keep your locks shiny, manageable, and young-looking, you need to make sure that they get enough moisture. This hot-oil hair treatment and in-shower scalp massage will work wonders.

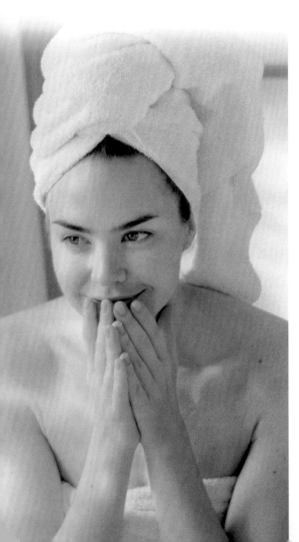

CARDAMOM HOT-OIL HAIR TREATMENT

Work this treatment into dry hair for best results.

1 Pour enough boiling water to fill a medium heatproof bowl halfway.

2 Pour two tablespoons of jojoba carrier oil into a smaller heatproof dish. Add six drops of cardamom essential oil and stir in.

3 Place the small dish in the medium one, resting it in the boiling water to warm the oil. Let stand for 5–10 minutes, then scoop the warm, fragrant oil into your hands and work it into your dry hair and scalp.

4 When your whole head is covered, take a large piece of plastic wrap and wrap your hair up in it like a turban. Wrap a warm towel around your head to finish, then sit comfortably and relax for 15 minutes.

5 Unwrap your head carefully. Take some shampoo and work it straight into your hair. Don't put water on before or with the shampoo, otherwise it will be very hard to get the oil out. When you have worked up a rich lather, get in the shower and rinse it all away.

LEFT You can make your hair look years younger by applying this treatment on a regular basis.

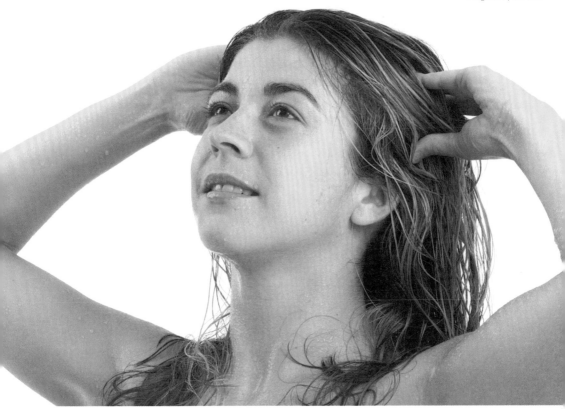

IN-SHOWER SCALP MASSAGE
This feels heavenly and will help to stimulate the hair follicles too, so your hair grows strong and healthy.

1 Lather your hair with a nourishing shampoo, then, while the shampoo is still on your hair, place both hands on either side of your head with your fingers above your ears.

2 Apply pressure in tiny, firm, circular movements with all your fingertips, then move up slightly and repeat.

3 Keep going until you have covered your whole head—your fingers will meet in the middle of your scalp. Repeat this process at least twice.

ABOVE Massaging your scalp feels great and will benefit more than just your hair—it's good for your circulation, too.

181

82

Protect yourself from the sun

The harmful UV rays of the sun are some of the most powerful and damaging aging agents in nature. However, you can still enjoy some time in the glorious sunshine and stay safe at the same time if you get sun-savvy with these top tips. They will keep you looking younger for longer as well!

BELOW A suntan looks good, but unfortunately it is seldom safe. Use a strong protection sunscreen at all times.

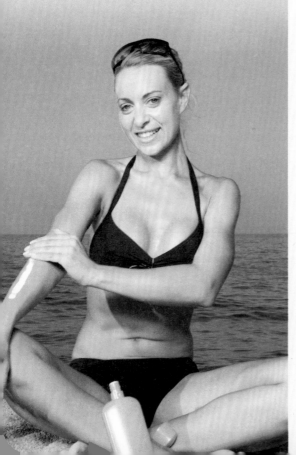

STAY SAFE IN THE SUN

- Always stay out of the sun when it's at its hottest, between 11 a.m. and 3 p.m.
- Cover up with a long-sleeved cotton kaftan and a wide-brimmed sun hat.
- Protect your eyes with dark sunglasses—be sure that they will filter out UVA-UVB rays.
- Never go out without using a sunscreen with a high SPF (of at least 15), and remember to reapply often if you are dipping in and out of the water or toweling yourself dry.
- Stay well hydrated by drinking a lot of fresh water throughout the day—aim for eight glasses, or the equivalent of two quarts.
- If you want to doze on a sunbed, make sure that you are in the shade and that someone is keeping an eye out and will wake you if the sun moves around so that you are in full sun.
- Don't be tricked by cloudy weather—the sun can still be very powerful.

If you do get burned, get out of the sun immediately and apply a cooling after-sun lotion. If you think you may have heatstroke, which occurs when the body is unable to control its temperature due to excessive heat, you must get to a doctor right away for treatment (symptoms include headaches, dizziness, nausea and vomiting, muscle pain, stomach cramps, tiredness, loss of appetite, and a high temperature).

Get the sun-kissed look

Sun and skincare experts agree that the only safe tan to have is one that comes out of a bottle. With skin cancer on the rise, it certainly pays to fake it. The good news is that modern formulations are really easy to apply and they create a fantastic result—it couldn't be easier to get glowing.

83

FAKE IT

The best thing about having a fake tan is that it makes you appear slimmer and more toned. In addition, it helps to "hide" cellulite. You should choose a formulation that develops overnight but which you can build up over time. Depending on your personal preference, you can opt for a cream/lotion, a mousse, or a clear spray.

Make sure you thoroughly moisturize your skin beforehand, because it will help you to get an even result and avoid streaking. Spend time massaging the product into your skin, and make sure you cover every inch. Apply liberally to legs, arms, chest, and shoulders, and use any excess on your hands to wipe over elbows, knees, and feet. Ask a friend to help cover your back and, when you're done, make sure you tissue off any excess product that's between your fingers and on your palms. You might want to use a separate formula on your face.

It's wise to let it dry for at least ten minutes before getting dressed, otherwise the tan may stain your clothes. Most fake tanning products take 12 hours to develop, so it's a good idea to apply it in the evening. That way, you can have a shower in the morning, which will also get rid of the distinctive smell that some products create. Build your color up over a few days or weeks until you are happy.

BELOW A suntan out of a bottle may not be the real thing, but it will look like the real thing and will keep you younger as well.

05

Young on the inside

While, of course, looking young is great, feeling young inside is just as important. Your emotional and spiritual well-being have a direct bearing on the way that you look, and taking care of the mind/body balance is key to a long, happy, and healthy life. This chapter offers a mix of soothing therapies and treatments with advice about how to sleep better and boost your energy, positive thinking, making time for yourself and embracing your inner strength.

Introduction

Happiness is a state of mind, not a physical actuality. How you respond to the environment around you and your experiences in it is what defines how you are feeling. The mind/body interaction is key to this process, and in order for your body to feel and look its youngest and healthiest, your mind must do the same.

YOUNG AT HEART, YOUNG IN MIND

Have you ever watched a very old man or woman grinning and dancing around like a teenager at a wedding or a party? Ever wondered how they do it? You might think they were "young at heart," as the old saying goes, but in fact as much as anything they would most likely be "young in mind." Of course, you need to have the physical capacity to be able to leap about enthusiastically in old age, but equally you must have the inclination—the mental energy and urge—to want to do so. Your mind could easily tell you not to do such a thing—you might injure yourself, it could be tiring—but while this is cautious and possibly prudent thinking, it is essentially negative thinking. Surely it is better to think "I could do that!" or "That would be fun!" and then leap up and start dancing, while, of course, being mindful of any physical impediments or disadvantages that might make you think twice about such an action? This is where the mind/body balance comes in—it's all about feeling young on the inside.

THE KEY TO ETERNAL YOUTH

You will age and you can't stop the process—but you can consciously decide how you are going to respond to it. By training your mind through meditation, positive visualization, and other techniques, combined with the assistance of relaxing and soothing physical therapies, such as yoga, reflexology, and massage, you can make the years fall off you—metaphorically, at least. Follow the detailed advice in this chapter, as well as these basic rules of engagement, and you will be young on the inside for evermore:

- Be open to new experiences—as we get older, we often become more cautious and fearful. Don't be; open up and embrace all that life has to offer.
- Celebrate your age—and the "experience" that comes with it. You have a lot to offer the world and everyone you know in it!
- Continue (or start) taking risks—you will get far more out of life if you do.
- Get yourself out there—be sociable and interact with people—it will do you good by improving your self-esteem and altering your perspective.
- Don't judge yourself or others solely by their age—it's only a number.

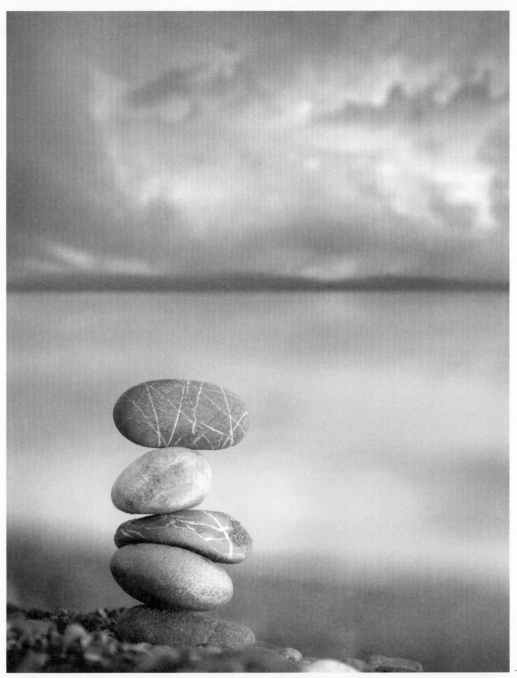

84

Balance your body and mind

Earlier in this book we looked at eating and drinking detox treatments for sustained youthfulness. Exercise and beauty programs complement the detox process, because they promote circulation, sweating, deep breathing, and flexibility. On an emotional level, they help to foster a sense of restoration and renewal.

BELOW & OPPOSITE
Achieving a healthy mind/ body balance is about keeping your whole self happy. It is never too late to work on your physical fitness and spiritual well-being.

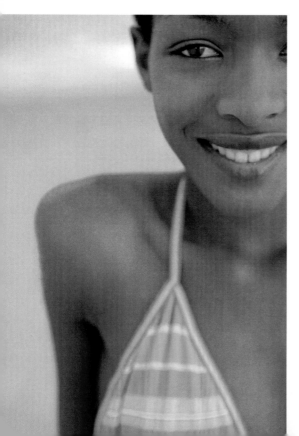

DETOX YOUR BODY

You can greatly enhance your vitality and general sense of well-being through a daily body care routine that you can easily carry out at home. Specific body treatments, from home spa therapies and natural hair and skin products to foot massage and aromatherapy, will leave you feeling pampered and nurtured, as well as significantly improving the appearance of your skin and the efficiency of your body's elimination processes. This book is full of these treatments and therapies, and any number of different combinations of the 100 ways to stay young proposed in this book will achieve the desired result.

Regular exercise is essential, not just for detoxing your body but for a happy, healthy life and to keep the mind/body balance in equilibrium at all times. Apart from stimulating sweating, improving general metabolism, and overall detoxification, exercise increases your self-esteem, reduces stress, and makes your body work more efficiently.

If exercise is something you normally avoid, read Chapter 2 again to find out why it is so important. And don't forget that exercise should be a pleasure rather than a chore. Exercise increases the production of free radicals in your body, so it must be accompanied by drinking sufficient fluids and the intake of antioxidant foods or supplements.

DETOX YOUR MIND

Many of the proposed tips and treatments in this book also explore some of the various complementary therapies that abound to help promote good health and well-being, primarily through reducing stress levels. Stress has disastrous effects on your health—it affects how your body works and causes the production of harmful toxins. In the course of this chapter, you will be shown how to reduce stress, detox your mind, and restore your inner harmony through a series of simple exercises, using tools such as meditation and visualization. Resting, relaxation, and recharging are also important for detoxing. Relaxation exercises help your body rebalance and prevent negative thoughts from interfering with the body's natural processes.

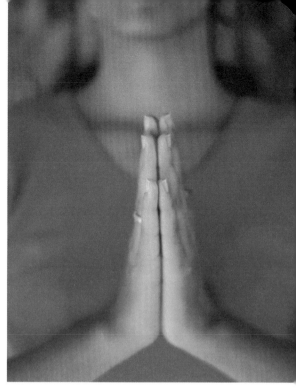

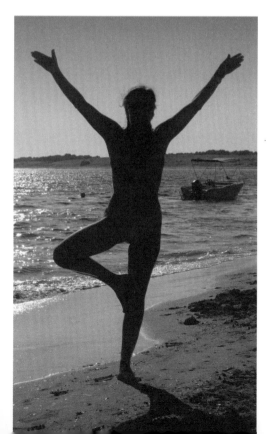

85

Massage for your body & soul

Therapeutic massage is an ancient technique used to promote general well-being and enhance self-esteem, while boosting the circulatory and lymphatic systems and reducing tension. Performed regularly by an expert practitioner, it is a superb destressing and antiaging tool that will make you feel great.

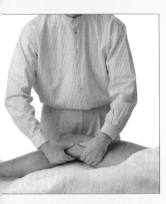

THE BENEFITS OF MASSAGE
Massage improves the supply of oxygen and nutrients to body tissues, enhances skin tone, and increases the elimination of chemical wastes from the body. At the same time it is an agreeable and soothing experience.

DIFFERENT TYPES OF MASSAGE
There are numerous kinds of massage, many of which have been incorporated into a variety of complementary therapies, but for detoxing and general antiaging purposes, aromatherapy massage and therapeutic massage are the best. You can massage yourself, although it is not as relaxing as being massaged by somebody else.

ABOVE Effleurage is a good, gentle technique with which to begin the massage.

FULL BODY MASSAGE
During a full body massage, which lasts about an hour, the practitioner will use a light vegetable oil or talcum powder to enable their hands to glide over the skin. Most strokes are carried out slowly and rhythmically toward the heart to help increase the blood and lymph circulation.

BASIC TECHNIQUES
Effleurage (stroking) is a gentle action for all parts of the body to warm and relax the muscles and aid circulation. Kneading techniques stretch and tone muscles. Pétrissage is similar to kneading in effect, but involves just using the thumbs and fingertips. Wringing, using the whole hand, is used on larger areas of the body. Percussion techniques, including tapotement, involve hacking with the sides of the hands to deliver short, sharp taps on the body.

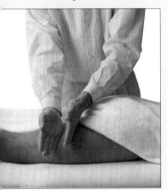

ABOVE Tapotement—a basic percussion technique—invigorates muscles and circulation.

OPPOSITE A massage of any kind will make you feel great, but one involving aromatherapy or therapeutic techniques is best for staying young.

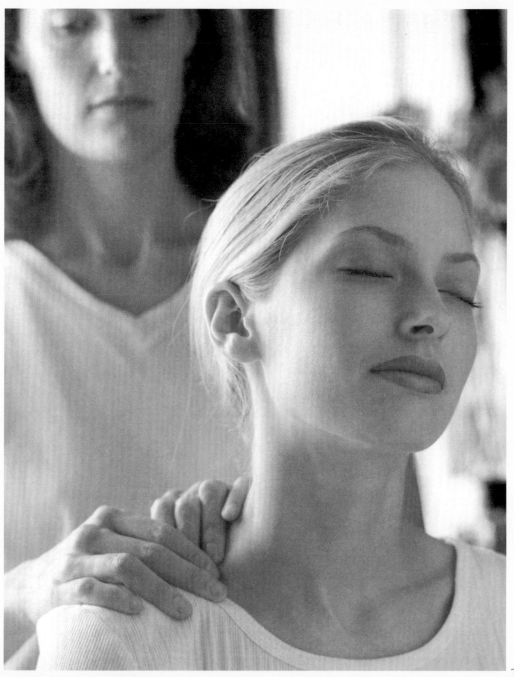

Aromatherapy treatments

Aromatherapy uses aromatic essential oils extracted from herbs, flowers, fruits, and trees. The oils are thought to penetrate the skin and travel through the body via the bloodstream and lymph vessels. Treatments with these natural oils are both immensely pleasurable and revivifying.

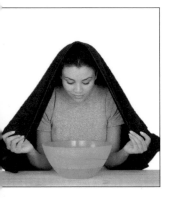

POINTS TO BEAR IN MIND

Aromatherapy oils are extremely potent and should not be applied directly to the skin or taken internally, and many oils are not suitable for use during pregnancy.

Essential oils are diluted in a vegetable-base carrier oil, such as almond or grapeseed oil, or blended in a lotion or cream. A normal dilution is six drops of essential oil (or a combination of up to three different oils) per 4 teaspoons of carrier oil, which is sufficient for a full body massage.

BASIC TECHNIQUES

- **Massage** Diluted as above.

ABOVE & BELOW You can inhale drops of aromatherapy oils, made from a variety of beneficial plants, from a bowl of steaming water.

- **Bathing** Add to bathwater, breaking up the oil on the surface to prevent it from burning the skin.

- **Steam inhalation** Add two to three drops of oil to a bowl of steaming hot water, lean your face over the bowl, drape a towel over your head, and breathe in the steam for a few minutes.

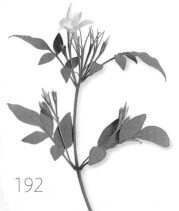

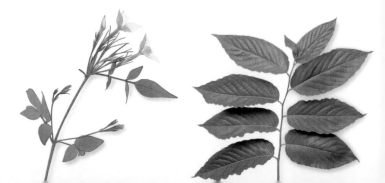

KEY DETOX OILS

Ten key oils for body detox
Basil
Fennel
Juniper
Lemon
Mandarin
Marjoram
Peppermint
Pine
Rose
Rosemary

Ten key oils for mind detox
Atlas cedarwood
Camomile
Eucalyptus
Geranium
Jasmine
Lavender
Lemon balm
Lime
Rose
Ylang-ylang

87

Detox your life

Following a short detox program will give your body a break from its toxic load and leave you feeling refreshed, invigorated, and ready for action. It should include all the elements of detoxing to enable your body to get rid of waste products more effectively and improve your underlying health.

BELOW Creating a soothing and relaxing environment will help your detox program to be successful.

CREATE A HOME HEALTH FARM

It's also all about pampering yourself from top to toe. A trip to a health farm can be an expensive luxury, but with a little planning you can easily create your own health farm at home where you can detox for the weekend.

WHAT SHOULD BE IN THE PROGRAM

A program of light eating that incorporates juices to stimulate the cleansing organs of the body, as well as giving your digestive system a rest, will serve as a good start. Other elements might include various treatments, such as aromatherapy, massage, and body scrubs, designed to help the detox process as well as making you feel and look good. You will also need to exercise to make your body function more efficiently and to help the elimination process. A spiritual element might incorporate meditation and visualization to help you detox your mind and induce inner harmony.

ENVIRONMENT

Before you start, make sure that your house is clean and tidy—or at least the rooms you will be using—so that you are not distracted by the need to do housework. Your bedsheets should be clean and fresh, as should your nightwear/leisurewear and robe. Turn the heating up a notch because you will be sitting around in loose clothing.

EQUIPMENT

The following items should help you relax thoroughly and keep you occupied during your detox routine:
- Selection of reading material (none of it should be work-related).
- Notepad or diary and something to write with.
- Art materials—raid your children's supplies for paper, pencils, or crayons, paints or modeling clay, or treat yourself to a cheap kit.
- Rug or duvet.

CREATING A HOME SPA

Turn your bathroom into a luxurious sanctuary so that you can feel relaxed and rejuvenated.

• Have large, thick cotton bath towels and soft washcloths available.

• Install some aromatherapy candles.

• Combine almond oil with a few drops of your favorite essential oil. Store in a decorative glass container and add to bathwater.

• Have an exfoliating scrub, face mask, loofah, and moisturizer available.

• A lot of pillows.
• Essential oils for relaxation—lavender, rose, or jasmine.
• Candles.
• Music to relax to or a relaxation tape.

FOOD

Try these basic foods and drinks to purify your system yet keep you properly nourished as you embark on your program:
• Variety of fresh fruit and vegetables.
• Herbal teas and filtered or bottled water.
• Olive oil.
• Selection of nuts and seeds.
• Goat milk yogurt.
• Brown rice.
• Fresh herbs.

88

Reflexology

Hand and foot massage have long been used to promote relaxation and improve health. The techniques involved in reflexology improve circulation and increase the efficiency of the rest of the body. The practice is long believed to have offered antiaging benefits.

THE PRINCIPLES OF REFLEXOLOGY

Practitioners of reflexology believe that the feet and hands are mirrors of the whole body and that pressure placed on specific reflex points on them can be used to treat the corresponding areas of the body, promoting well-being and stimulating the body's natural healing powers.

HOW DOES REFLEXOLOGY WORK?

Reflexology is a good complementary therapy for detoxing the body and the mind. Massaging the feet allows blood to circulate more freely, distributing oxygen and nutrients through the body and removing waste products.

THE BENEFITS OF REFLEXOLOGY

Reflexology can help your body detox by encouraging the organs of elimination to work well. Stimulating the reflex points is thought to help eliminate waste products, which are felt as tender granular or crystalline deposits in the feet or hands. The aim is to break down these deposits and improve the blood supply to flush away toxins. Specific reflex points to work on while detoxing include the spleen/pancreas, stomach, adrenal glands, colon, liver, gallbladder, and kidneys.

BASIC TECHNIQUES

Practitioners usually work with the feet because they are more sensitive. The practitioner gives an initial massage to relax the feet and then massages the whole of each foot to stimulate the reflex points. Extra massage is given to break down crystalline deposits and free energy flow. The practitioner will use the pad of the thumb to move over the skin, applying and releasing pressure before creeping along slightly and repeating the action. You can practice reflexology on your own hands or feet, although you will benefit more from a professional treatment.

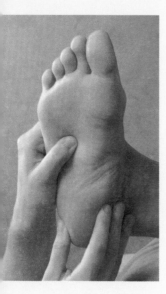

ABOVE The practitioner will begin with a gentle warm-up massage to relax the feet.

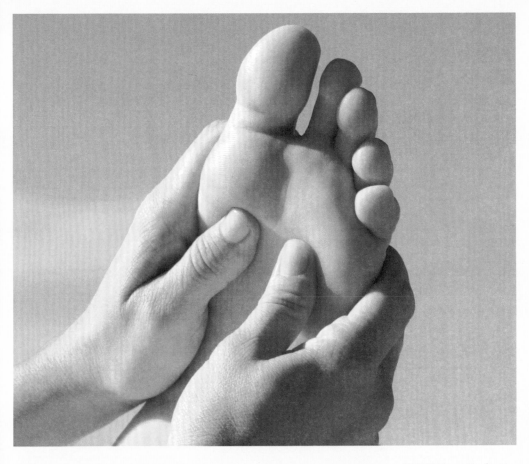

ABOVE The entire foot is carefully massaged, with the pads of the thumbs doing most of the work.

DO-IT-YOURSELF REFLEXOLOGY TECHNIQUES

The foot roll is an excellent beginner's technique that you can practice on yourself, your partner, or friend. It is a good way to pick up the basic manipulations that other reflexology techniques require.

• Place your palms on either side of the foot and roll the foot between your hands.

• To create the rolling motion of the foot, move each hand in opposite directions.

• Start slowly and then roll faster.

197

89

Practice yoga

Practiced for thousands of years, yoga was originally developed as a system of mental and physical training in preparation for spiritual growth. It is a great way of keeping the aging process at bay and is as popular now as it has ever been. Build it into your daily program and feel rapid benefits.

TYPES OF YOGA

There are many types of yoga, all of which incorporate various asanas (postures) and breathing techniques. Yoga enables you to cultivate a fit and flexible body as well as a balanced mind and emotions.

THE BENEFITS OF YOGA

Various yoga postures can be extremely helpful for detoxing because they stimulate the digestion and lymphatic system. Others improve circulation and increase the supply of oxygen. Everyone, regardless of age or fitness level, can benefit from yoga.

BASIC TECHNIQUES

It is very important to join a yoga class or take lessons from a qualified practitioner. After guiding you through some gentle warm-up exercises, your teacher will show you the correct way to perform yoga postures, which you then practice with the rest of the class, followed by a period of relaxation.

ABOVE The classic yoga pose, Warrior II.

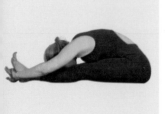

ABOVE Some yoga poses require a lot of practice and flexibility, such as this sitting stretch.

TOP FIVE YOGA HINTS FOR BEGINNERS

1 **Always use a proper yoga mat, because there is a real risk of slipping on any other surface.**

2 **Create a relaxing atmosphere. Light a candle or burn some incense.**

3 **To start with, set yourself a goal to practice yoga for 20–25 minutes daily.**

4 **Consult your doctor before you begin to practice yoga.**

5 **Try to stay in the present moment. Don't let your mind wander, because it might distract you.**

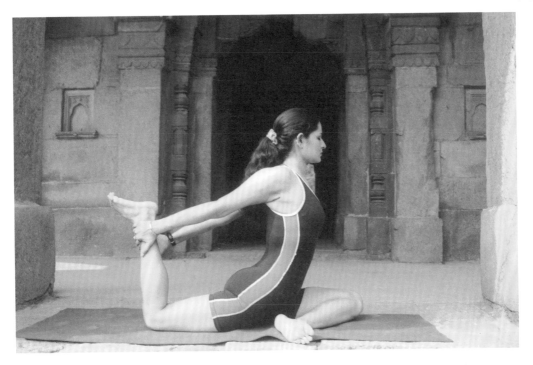

TAKE IT SLOWLY

When practicing yoga by yourself, you should progress gradually and never force your body into postures before you are ready. Aim to practice for at least 20 minutes daily to increase your energy and stamina, tone muscles, improve digestion, help you deal with stress, and improve concentration. Allow at least two hours after a meal before exercising. Seek medical advice before doing upside-down poses, such as shoulder stands, if you have any physical problems affecting your heart, neck, blood pressure, ears, or eyes.

ABOVE Yoga is a very ancient Asian art, with many associations. Some of the poses are designed to replicate animals, plants, and other elements from the natural world.

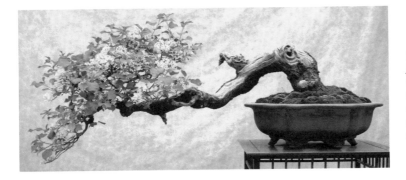

LEFT The ancient Japanese tree sculpting art of bonsai has close links with yoga and other Asian arts designed to promote spiritual growth and contemplation.

199

90

Think positively

Positive thinking is the ability to consider things in an optimistic, upbeat manner—to think with a "can do" attitude. Used effectively, its power is immense and the value of a positive mental attitude is priceless—especially as you become older. Aspire to positive thinking, whatever your age.

HOW TO THINK POSITIVELY

If you have spent your life thinking in negative patterns—believing that things are not possible, or that things will go wrong—it can be hard to change these ingrained attitudes. Perhaps you have good reason to think in that way; after all, we are all products of what life throws at us down the years. However, a habit of positive thinking can be cultivated at any age and at any pass in your life—it just takes a little practice. Try these ten practical tips for positive thinking and see if you can change the way you look at the world. If you can successfully apply them, they will enhance your life and make you feel younger.

1 Find good role models It is said that you become what you think about all day. Associate yourself with people who think positively and learn from them.

2 Think "glass half full," not "half empty" Be optimistic in your assessment of what happens to you in your everyday life. There will be better days. Belief and hope are half the battle.

3 Don't allow negative emotions to overwhelm you You might have had a really bad day or a bad experience—but it's not the end of the world! Live to fight another day. Stand up and fight. See the good in any bad situation.

4 Be thankful Whatever happens, there are worse situations. However you are feeling, there is someone worse off than yourself. Be grateful for your life and good fortune. Gratitude unlocks other positive feelings and calms and expands the mind.

5 Believe Even if everything tells you otherwise, trust your gut feeling. Believe that things can improve, that life will become better. If you think positively enough, it surely will.

6 Persist Push yourself on toward your goal. You might have been knocked back a hundred times already, but keep going. Persevere and you will get there in the end. Don't give up.

7 Take responsibility instead of blaming Learn to acknowledge if a fault or failing is of your own making, as opposed to blaming someone else. If you take charge of your feelings and behavior and responsibility for your actions, you will feel better about yourself—and everyone else will feel better about you.

8 Look to alternative sources of help Don't rely on your "default" settings—look somewhere new for help and guidance. If you are religious, pray and consult your divinity.

9 Don't give up on your dreams Accept your situation when you have to, but never stop believing that something better might be waiting just around the corner.

10 Keep the big picture in mind Distractions, pettiness—they can irritate you for a moment, but never lose sight of who you are, what you are here for, and what you are trying to achieve. Don't concentrate too much on the details in life—successful living is about the bigger picture.

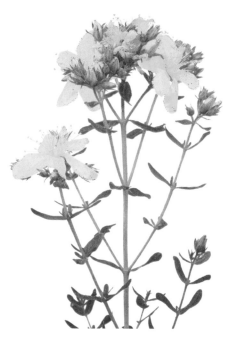

OPPOSITE Positive thinking can have wonderful—and rapid—all-around effects. If used consistently and effectively, it could change your whole approach to your life.

ABOVE St. John's Wort (Hypericon) has for centuries been used as a natural remedy to promote positive thought. If you are struggling for a positive frame of mind, try it in extract form.

✳ **TIP BOX**

A CREDO FOR LIFE
Positive thinking is more than simply looking on the "bright side." It is an entire lifestyle of thinking rightly, which will leave you more fulfilled, happy, and satisfied than ever before. It doesn't matter how old you are when you come to realize its benefits.

91

Neurolinguistic programing

Neurolinguistic programing (NLP) is an approach to psychotherapy that is based on the principle that patterns of thought and behavior and the subjective experiences underlying them can be fundamentally changed. It is something that could make you feel younger if it works for you.

WHAT IS NLP?

NLP is a relatively new system of alternative therapy that seeks to educate people in self-awareness and effective communication and to change their patterns of mental and emotional behavior. The cofounders of the therapy, Richard Bandler and linguist John Grinder, believed that NLP would be useful in "finding ways to help people have better, fuller, and richer lives." They coined the term "NeuroLinguistic Programing" (NLP) to emphasize their belief in a connection between the neurological processes ("neuro"), language ("linguistic"), and behavioral patterns that have been learned through experience ("programing") and can be organized to achieve specific goals in life.

HOW DOES NLP HELP YOU FEEL YOUNGER?

Practitioners of NLP claim that it works incredibly quickly and can rejuvenate a person's general attitude and behavior far more rapidly than conventional forms of therapy. In NLP, there is a particular emphasis on phobias and how to overcome them. The founders of the therapy believe that deep-seated fears and phobias are primarily responsible for holding people back in their lives and that overcoming them through essential changes of mindset is the key to feeling better—and possibly even younger, into the bargain.

THE SUCCESS OF NLP

There are countless books and web sites devoted to NLP and courses in the therapy are widely available. One of the reasons for its huge popularity is that NLP claims to be capable of addressing the full range of problems that psychologists are likely to encounter, including depression, habit disorder, psychosomatic illnesses, and learning disorders, as well as phobias. It also espouses the potential for self-determination through overcoming learned limitations and emphasizes well-being and healthy functioning. NLP has also been promoted as a "science of excellence," derived from the study of how high achievers in different fields obtain their results.

***TIP BOX**

COMPLEMENTARY THERAPIES
NLP is a good stand-alone therapy that works for many people, but is also flexible enough to be used in conjunction with the many other therapies and treatments covered in this book.

OPPOSITE NLP aims to train your mind and behavior much as a professional musician is trained to perform—by emulating excellence in tried and tested techniques.

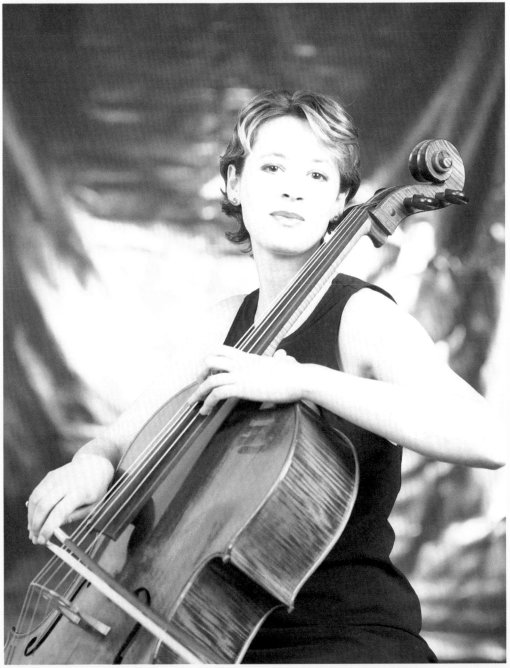

92

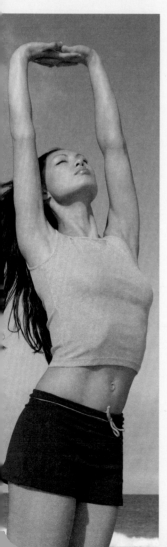

Be an optimist

An optimist is someone who generally believes that good things are going to happen. Optimists enjoy many health and lifestyle benefits, and tend to be happier than other people overall. Being optimistic will probably make you feel younger and healthier, also, although this is hard to quantify.

HOW IS OPTIMISM DEFINED?

Optimism is measured by your personal explanatory style, or how you define events. If you can learn to define positive events as being:

- because of something you did
- a sign of more good things to come
- evidence that good things will happen in other areas of your life

... then you are a long way toward being an optimist. If you can also think of negative events as:

- not your fault
- isolated occurrences that have no bearing on future events or other areas of your life

... then you are the rest of the way there!

ARE YOU AN OPTIMIST?

Consider the following questions and statements carefully to find out if you are an optimist:

1 **When something positive happens** in your life, stop to analyze your thought process for a moment. Are you giving yourself due credit for making it happen? Think of all the strengths you possess and the ways that you contributed, both directly and indirectly, to make this event occur. For example, if you did well in an examination or test of some kind, don't just think of how great it is that you were prepared, but also think of how your intelligence and dedication played a role in your success.

2 **Think of other areas of your life** that could be affected by this good event. Also, think of how the strengths you possess that caused this good thing to happen can also cause other positive events in your life.

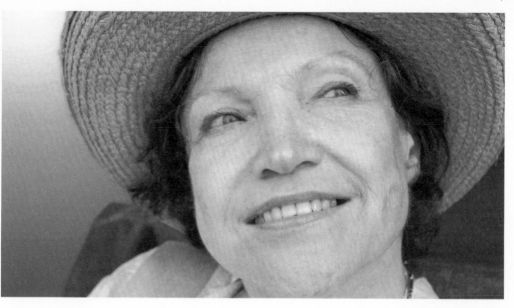

3 **Imagine what future possibilities** could be in store. Because you hold the key to your success, shouldn't you expect to do well on future tests?

4 **When negative events occur,** think of the extenuating circumstances that could have contributed to them happening. If you didn't do well on an exam, for example, were you especially busy in the preceding week?

5 **Also remember** that you'll have endless opportunities to do better in the future. Concentrate on your next potential success.

OPPOSITE & ABOVE It is not always easy for all of us, but if you can think like an optimist and believe that it is all good, you will feel younger and happier.

TOP HINTS FOR BECOMING AN OPTIMIST

• The key to optimism is to maximize your successes and minimize your failures.

• It is beneficial to look honestly at your shortcomings so you can work on them, but focusing on your strengths can never hurt.

• Bear in mind that the more you practice challenging your thought patterns, the more automatic the process will become.

• Practice positive affirmations. They really work!

Embrace your inner strength

Life is not always easy and things can go wrong at any point. There are times when you must reach inside yourself to find inner strength in order to cope with what you are facing. This might involve thinking back to an earlier, happier time in your life, which of itself could help you feel rejuvenated and more positive.

COPING WITH A HARD TIME

Are you feeling down and drained? Well, the good news is that it is a lot easier than you might think to boost your inner strength and pick yourself up. By boosting your inner strength, you can change your life for the better and feel younger and more optimistic about everything. Try these ten simple steps to see if you can boost your inner strength. All you need is an open mind and a willingness to try.

1 **Make a list of your successes** each night before you go to sleep in bed— no matter how small or insignificant they might seem to be. This activity will prime your brain to tune in to more success in the future.

2 **Positive affirmations are a great way** of embracing your inner strength. Repeat phrases, such as "I am strong and healthy." "I believe in myself." Studies have shown that positive affirmations improve focus and boost your resolution to get things done.

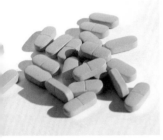

ABOVE & BELOW
Vitamins and spiritual reflection will both help you find inner strength in very different ways.

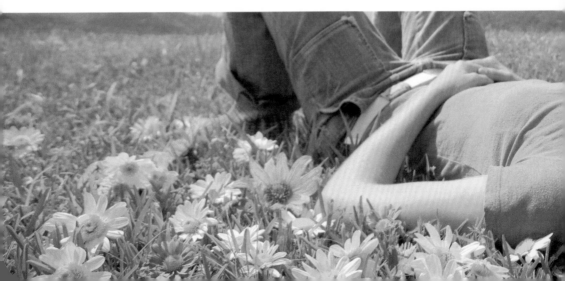

3 **Reconnect with your friends.** Having friends who support you will give you strength. Even a quick chat with a friend will remind you that you are not alone.

4 **Spending time with your pet** has been proven to improve your inner strength. Apparently, interaction with animals we are close to releases hormones that make our bodies feel stronger.

5 **Focus on your spiritual connection.** If you are religious, pray and ask for inner strength.

6 **Take daily vitamins and minerals.** Drink water throughout the day instead of coffee and soft drinks. Take vitamin and mineral supplements to improve your well-being. Feeling better physically will boost your inner strength.

7 **Laugh as much as possible.** Laughing releases endorphins and positive hormones that will make you feel better about everything.

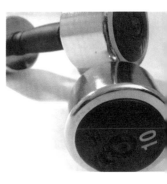

8 **Turn to your partner.** Ask them to listen, tell them how you are feeling, and then bask in the warmth of their love and support.

9 **Keep a small pair of weights in your home.** Lift them with your arms and do knee bends throughout the day for a few minutes at a time whenever you have a few moments. Stretch your muscles out as much as you can, because this will increase blood flow and improve circulation, making you feel better.

10 **Avoid as much television as possible.** Instead, do some gardening or indulge in some other kind of healthy hobby that you enjoy.

ABOVE The most gentle of workouts with light weights in your armchair will release endorphins and improve blood flow.

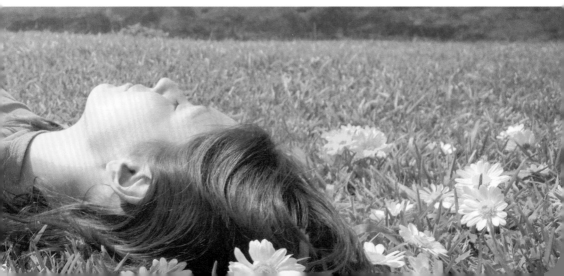

Make time for yourself

With greater age comes greater responsibilities, and it can be easy to lose sight of yourself and your personal desires as you constantly look after others and take care of their needs. However, part of staying young involves pampering yourself regularly and ensuring that your own requirements for time and space are met.

STRESS AND GUILT

If you are a busy mom with several children—and maybe a job as well—you will know what it feels like never to have enough time to do everything you think you should be doing. The daily round of essential chores and responsibilities can be wearing enough in itself, but over a period of time it can be accompanied by negative feelings of guilt and inadequacy that are stressful and can make you feel even worse about things. If you are stressed, you might feel that you are not doing enough for your children or others—or doing it in the right way. This can lead to a destructive and dangerous cycle in your behavior, which means that you try ever harder while putting more and more pressure on yourself and not allowing yourself enough time to relax and have some "me" time.

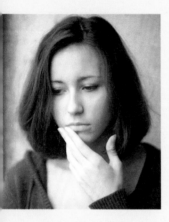

ABOVE Don't take everything on your own shoulders all the time. You are entitled to quality time off for yourself—just like everyone else.

Does this sound like you? Everyone deserves some time to themselves—and that includes you, so don't feel guilty. Besides, time out can be energizing and rejuvenating, enabling you later on to pick up where you left off with renewed vigor. Try these few ideas for how to make time for yourself and what to do with it:

- Record your thoughts and feelings in a diary. This could be a good starting point to understanding why you so often neglect yourself and your own needs.
- Pamper yourself with a relaxing soak in the bathtub.
- Curl up and read a favorite book.
- Chill out in the yard with a long, cool drink and a magazine.
- Go window shopping, or treat yourself to those clothes or that DVD that you have had your eye on.
- Do some exercise, or lose yourself in your favorite hobby. Exercising will help drive out stress hormones and will make you feel better.
- Remind yourself that your own life is just as important as those of others.

Live more simply

Are you happy with your life? As you become older, is it matching up to your expectations? If the answer to these questions is "no," perhaps you have lost sight of the basic pleasure of existence. You might benefit from simplifying your life a little and getting back in touch with nature.

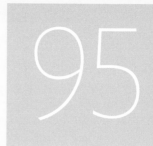

THE PRESSURES OF MODERN LIFE

Nowadays we all live such hectic, fast-paced lives. This is wearing and prematurely aging. But does it have to be this way? Is this the only way to live? Sometimes, just "being," in the moment of your existence, can be a real eye-opener and can rejuvenate and make you feel more positive about your experience of day-to-day living. Try these easy tips to make your life simpler:

- Stop and smell the flowers—next time you are outside, do just that.
- Close your eyes and listen—appreciate the sounds of nature.
- Watch nature at work—observe a bird twittering or a squirrel in a tree.
- Reach out and touch—caress the bud of a tree or an ear of corn.
- Breathe deeply and feel the rhythm of the natural world.

BELOW Modern life can be tough and demanding. Sometimes a return to the simple things—to nature—can be hugely beneficial and therapeutic.

96

Promote good chi

The ancient Chinese art of Feng Shui—pronounced "fung shway" and translating as "wind and water"—is based on the principle of creating a positive environment in the home, or office, by obtaining a good flow of "chi"—the force of energy that the Chinese believe drives the universe.

THE CONTEMPORARY TAKE ON FENG SHUI

A somewhat "New Age," Western interpretation of this ancient Chinese art has become a popular way of making our homes and other surroundings a positive place in which to spend time and to live in harmony with our environment. There are many interesting but extremely complicated factors that are part of the Feng Shui way of living. However, there are also some good, simple ideas for improved health and greater youthfulness that are easier to incorporate into our lives and our homes.

Here are five simple tips for promoting better chi in your home and environment:

1 **Get rid of clutter.** Most clutter is negative. It disrupts the flow of chi, which is life energy. It is especially important to remove clutter from the center of your house, because this area is considered the heart and/or focus of the home. Other areas of the "bagua" (which is a Feng Shui map that divides your house into nine sections) are all touched by the center health area. This means all areas of your house are affected by what is in your health area and vice versa. This principle then applies to your life, because all areas of your life are affected by your health, and your health affects all parts of your life. Therefore, it is important to keep the center of your house clutter-free to allow positive energy, "qi," to flow throughout your home.

2 **Use the senses to your advantage in your home.** Balance and harmony in your home will both stabilize and energize you and your family. Use colors to create the appropriate mood. Red will keep you going—it's bright and full of energy—but do not use it in bedrooms if you want to rest. Orange is refreshing and revitalizing—use it in the kitchen or playrooms. Its softer

shades can be used in family rooms where it promotes fun and relaxation. Yellow is a happy color that promotes creativity and vitality. Use it in a kitchen or office. Green is a healing and calming color. It is great for living rooms or bedrooms, because it renews and keeps us in balance. Blue is also a healing color, as well as a mentally relaxing color. Add blue to a room when someone is sick—it will keep the room's occupants calm. Use natural lighting when possible, and dimmer switches to change the atmosphere from bright and energizing to low and calming as needed. Remember that touch is an important and often overlooked sense. Softness and warmth can be used to relax; rough textures and coolness will energize. Aromas are another way to vary or change the atmosphere or feeling of a room or an entire home. Essential oils, good-quality scented candles, and fresh air all promote the change of energy in your home.

BACKGROUND IMAGE
Japanese zen gardens—featuring perfectly spherical boulders and beautifully raked gravel—are based on the principles of feng shui.

3 **Improve the center of your home.** As stated earlier, the middle or heart of your house is associated with health. By adding live plants to this area, you will improve the energies that are required for good health and balance. Add yellow and earth tones to give your health chi a boost. By adding square shapes and flat items to this area, you will allow energetic movement, which the ancient Chinese believed is an aid to good health.

4 **Make changes or additions to your bedroom.**
The bedroom is where you spend a great deal of your time, so it is an important room for your health. Reducing electromagnetic fields is one of the best things you can do for better health. Remove all electrical appliances from the bedroom if possible. If not, place them at least two yards from the bed. Things like electric blankets or waterbeds are the worst offenders, due to their proximity to your body as you sleep.

5 **Place objects in certain areas of your home** for good health and for energizing you and your family. A model of a dragon is a good health symbol, but do not place it in the bedroom because it has too much energy and would make the bedroom restless instead of restive.

97

Boost your energy

Modern life is fast-paced, demanding, and relentless. It requires and depletes a lot of energy. If you want to partake of it to the full, you need to find ways of recharging your batteries in the face of a constant drain on your resources. The good news is that you will stay young in the process.

KEEPING UP APPEARANCES

Do you ever feel as though you are being left behind in life? Does its fast pace take its toll on you, particularly as you become older? Try these tips and techniques to boost your energy and stay young.

1 **Sleep at the right time.** Most of us know that eight hours of sleep per night is optimal. However, what many people don't know is that the actual time you fall asleep is important as well. Due to the 24-hour cycle that your body clock is governed by—the natural light exposure-triggered Circadian rhythm—sleeping from 1 a.m. to 9 a.m. is not thought to be as restorative as sleeping from 10 p.m. to 6 a.m. The later in the evening you fall asleep and the later in the morning you wake up, the more out-of-sync your cycle becomes. Consequently, try to go to bed before 10 p.m.

2 **Abdominal breathing.** In Chinese medicine, energy is called "qi" (pronounced "chi"), and one of the most important ways you make qi is by breathing deeply to the pit of your stomach. Stress, poor posture, and a straining waistline might be some of the reasons why your breath doesn't make it down to the bottom of your lungs. However, try abdominal breathing as a simple way of increasing your qi energy and improving your stamina.

3 **Eliminate energy-sapping foods from your diet.** Too much coffee and sugar and not enough water, protein, and alkaline-forming foods, such as green leafy vegetables, will sap your energy. Ditch high-sugar-content foods, caffeine, and alcohol and eat more good, healthy stuff.

4 **Take a stress-formula multivitamin.** People who are under chronic stress require more B vitamins than other people. A "stress formula" multivitamin preparation often contains more B vitamins than standard proprietary multivitamins.

OPPOSITE Gently working out with weights at home or in the gym is one good way of boosting your energy, but there are a lot of other less strenuous things you can do.

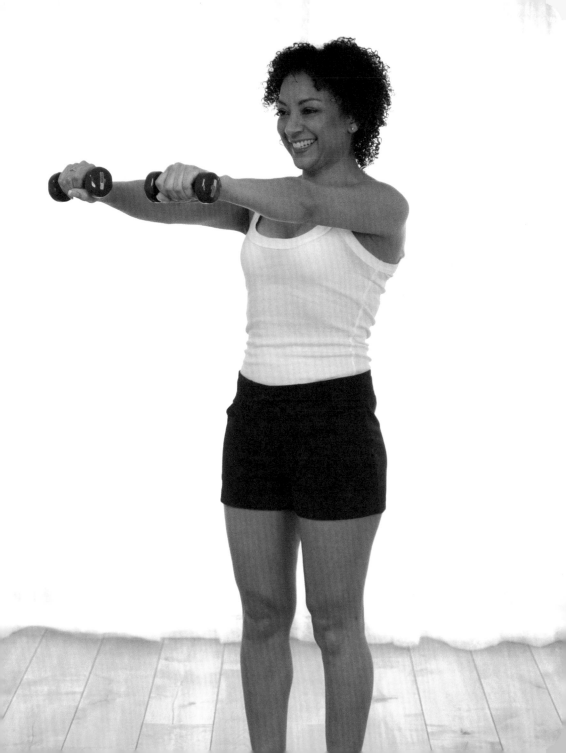

98

Get a great night's sleep

It is impossible to overestimate the benefits of a good night's sleep, whatever age you are. We all have different sleep needs, but the typical adult requires an average of at least seven and ideally eight hours per night. A healthy regime of nightly rest will keep you looking your best and feeling young.

ABOVE Circadian rhythms: Our bodies are programed to sleep at night when it is dark and the moon is shining.

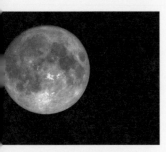

ABOVE Lighting a few scented candles that give off only a little light should help get you in the mood for sleep.

WHAT ARE THE BENEFITS?

The benefits of sleep are so numerous that entire books have been written on the subject! Here is a selection of the best.

- Sleep helps to repair your body—by allowing it to produce extra protein molecules.

- Sleep helps keep your heart healthy—by reducing the levels of stress and inflammation in your body.

- Sleep reduces stress—by helping to lower blood pressure and elevated levels of stress hormones.

- Sleep improves your memory—because, as you sleep, your brain is busy organizing and correlating memories.

- Sleep helps control body weight issues—by helping to regulate the hormones that affect and control your appetite.

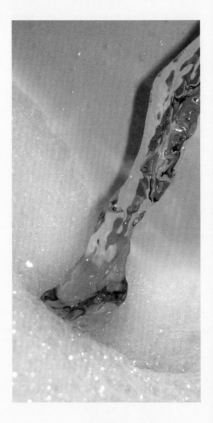

ABOVE If you have trouble getting off to sleep in the evenings, try a warm, foamy bath before bedtime.

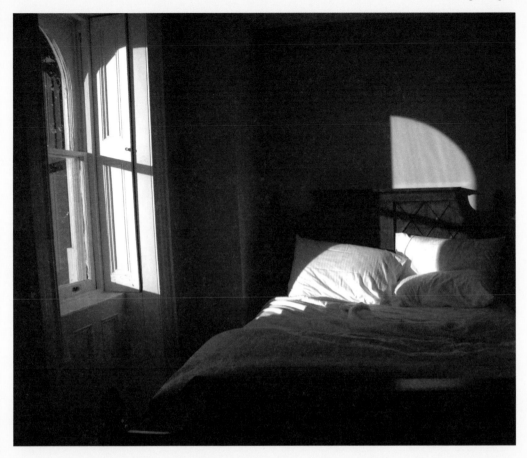

GOOD IDEAS FOR A GREAT NIGHT'S SLEEP

• Go to bed and get up at the same time every day.

• Never nap during the day, because this will confuse your body clock.

• Create a relaxing bedtime routine that works for you.

• Don't overeat before bedtime or go to bed hungry.

• Make your bedroom a haven of peace and tranquility.

ABOVE The darker you keep your bedroom at night, the easier you will find it to drift off to a good night's sleep.

Boost your self-esteem

As they become older and lose their looks and physical beauty, some people experience a drop in their self-esteem. This can be detrimental in many ways, and can even affect health. However, the good news is that there are a lot of ways of regaining self-esteem and feeling great about yourself once more.

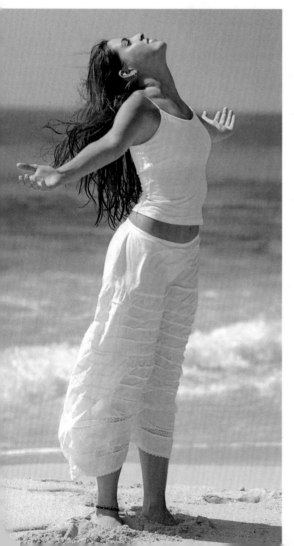

DO YOU LACK SELF-CONFIDENCE?

Hands up if you have a lack of self-confidence. There is nothing to be ashamed of—many people do. But what can you do about it? If you aren't happy with your life at the moment, don't worry, because you have the power to change it. Try the following suggestions to boost your self-confidence and self-esteem right away.

PROGRAM YOUR BRAIN

Did you know you can "program" your brain to boost your self-esteem? Think of it as a super-computer. Now, debug the system, throw away all the trash and keep only the "good" files.

- Start thinking positively.
- Congratulate yourself when things go right.

START THE DAY RIGHT

Put yourself in a positive frame of mind before you even get out of bed by asking yourself these questions:

- What am I happy about in my life?
- What am I excited about?
- Who do I love?
- Who loves me?

CULTIVATE YOUR SOCIAL LIFE

People with high self-esteem are generally sociable. As a rule, the more you interact with other people, the more positive you will feel about yourself. Join a voluntary organization or club and offer to help.

GET SOME EXERCISE
Include more exercise in your life. Working out, particularly outdoors, is a great way to generate your own "feel-good" chemicals and will give you body confidence as well as energize you.

RELAX
Do you spend a lot of time feeling anxious and stressed? Learning to breathe like a relaxed and confident person will help you cope with daily stresses, and it's easy to learn how.

REVIEW YOUR SITUATION
Include time for reflection in your daily schedule—praying if you are religious, meditating, or writing a diary of your thoughts and feelings.

CHANGE YOUR ENVIRONMENT
The chances are that your environment reflects the way you feel. However, whether it is dull, cluttered, or messy, you can change it. Any positive changes you make will have a positive effect on your mood as well.

GIVE YOURSELF A TREAT
Start treating yourself the way you would treat your best friend. Many people just aren't very nice to themselves a lot of the time. If this applies to you, try to change the situation by giving yourself encouragement and support.

FIND A ROLE MODEL
If you have difficulty taking this new, kinder version of yourself seriously, why not pretend to be someone else? Think of someone you admire—it might be someone you know, or someone famous—and live your day as you think they would.

100

Have fun, live long!

If you follow all the advice in this book—all 100 tips and more—then there is a good chance that you will stay younger for longer and live a happier and healthier life in the process. However, there is one thing that you can do that will help you in this quest more than anything else—enjoy your life.

LAUGHTER LINES

Laughter is good for you—it's official. Numerous studies have shown that the more you laugh the better you are likely to feel and the longer you will live. Nobody is quite sure why this is the case, although there is evidence that laughter releases positive hormones and endorphins in the brain and body, so that the reason for the resulting change in mood is primarily chemical. Do whatever makes you laugh and it will benefit you, as will the following tips:

- Drink red wine—red wine is packed with resveratrol, an antioxidant. This works to protect your body against the effects of aging. One or two glasses of red wine a day can help keep your body feeling young.

✳ TIP BOX

HAVE MORE SEX
Sex and touching are thought to be essential parts of health. Sex releases an assortment of beneficial chemicals in the body and helps us bond with others. Frequent sex may even extend your life by a number of years.

OPPOSITE Spending quality time with those you care most about will lift your spirits and benefit your health. Relax and enjoy life to the full!

- Eat dark chocolate—dark chocolate made from cocoa contains a large amount of antioxidants that protect your body from aging. Eating chocolate may lower your blood pressure and cholesterol while providing an energy boost.
- Relax—relaxation is the opposite of stress. While stress brings harmful health effects, relaxation helps our bodies to rest, heal, and function better.
- Turn exercise into play—physical games and sports are a great way to keep both your body and mind healthy. Simple exercise routines are excellent for maintaining balance, flexibility, endurance, and strength.
- Sleep—sleeping is an essential body function. The health benefits of sleep include more energy, better immune function, and more.

Useful addresses and web sites

If you are really serious about staying young and increasing your longevity as much as possible, there are lots of other practical measures you can take. The following organizations can offer you valuable help and assistance with specific areas of your health and anti-aging routine.

American Academy of Sleep Medicine—ASDA
One Westbrook Corporate Center,
Suite 920
Westchester, IL 60154
Organization URL(s):
inquiries@aasmnet.org
www.aasmnet.org/

American Heart Association
7272 Greenville Ave.
Dallas, TX 75231
Customer Service:
Tel: (800) AHA-USA-1
Tel: (800) 242-8721
Tel: (888) 474-VIVE
www.heart.org/HEARTORG/

American Herbalists Guild
PO Box 230741
Boston, MA 02123
Tel: (857) 350-3128
E-mail: ahgoffice@earthlink.net
www.americanherbalistsguild.com/

American Institute of Stress
The American Institute of Stress
124 Park Ave.
Yonkers, NY 10703
Tel: (914) 963-1200
Fax: (914) 965-6267
E-mail: Stress125@optonline.net
www.stress.org/

American Massage Therapy Association
500 Davis St.,
Suite 900
Evanston, IL 60201-4695
Tel: (847) 864-0123
Toll-free: (877)-905-0577
Fax: (847) 864-5196
E-mail: info@amtamassage.org
www.amtamassage.org

American Osteopathic Association
1090 Vermont Ave. NW, Suite 510
Washington, D.C. 20005-4949
Tel: (202) 414-0140
Toll-free: (800) 962-9008
Fax: (202) 544-3525

American Society for Nutrition
9650 Rockville Pike
Bethesda, MD 20814
Tel: (301) 634-7050
Fax: (301) 634-7892
www.nutrition.org/

The Council on Chiropractic Education
8049 N. 85th Way
Scottsdale, AZ 85258-4321
Tel: (480) 443-8877
Toll-free: (888) 443-3506
Fax: (480) 483-7333
E-mail: cce@cce-usa.org
www.cce-usa.org

National Association for Holistic Aromatherapy
PO BOX 1868
Banner Elk, NC 28604
Tel: (828) 898-6161
Fax: (828) 898-1965
www.naha.org/
E-mail: info@naha.org_

Yoga Alliance
1701 Clarendon Blvd.,
Suite 110
Arlington, VA 22209
Tel: (888) 921.YOGA (9642)
www.yogaalliance.org//

Index

Acknowledgments

The publishers would like to thank the following individuals and agencies for contributing copyright images to this book:

Colin Bowling: pp. 131, 135, 137, 168
Clive Bozzard-Hill: pp. 46, 47
Corbis: pp. 178, 179, 180, 181, 188
Digital Vision: p. 203
Focus Publishing: pp. 34, 35, 36, 37, 38, 39, 42, 45, 141 (top), 193
Getty Images: pp. 174-5, 204, 217
iStock: pp. 4, 6-7, 9, 10-11, 13, 17, 21, 43, 44, 59, 71, 123, 157, 158, 159, 160, 161, 162, 163, 165, 166, 167, 170, 171, 172, 173, 176, 177, 182, 183, 187, 200, 201, 207 (bottom), 208, 210-11, 216, 218-19
Ivy Press: pp. 26, 27, 66, 67
Trevor Leighton: pp. 130, 132, 133, 134, 136, 138, 139
Roddy Paine: p. 213
Ian Parsons: pp. 46, 47, 70-119, 124, 125, 126, 127, 140, 141, 142-9, 152, 153, 169, 213
Retna Pictures Ltd: pp. 65, 152
stock.xchng: pp. 18, 19, 20, 22, 23, 24, 25, 28, 29, 30, 31, 32-3, 40, 41, 54, 55, 68, 69, 189 (bottom), 197, 199, 205, 206, 207, 209, 214, 215
Calvey Taylor-Haw: pp. 48, 49, 50, 51, 52, 53, 60, 61, 62, 63, 189, 190, 191, 192, 194, 195, 196, 198